# The Road Trip

## Life with Autism

Gloria Pearson-Vasey
and
J. Kevin Vasey

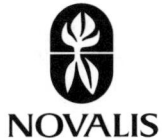

© 2005 Novalis, Saint Paul University, Ottawa, Canada

Cover design: Dominique Pelland
Cover image: Jupiter Images (photos.com)
Layout: Caroline Galhidi

Business Office:
Novalis
49 Front Street East, 2nd Floor
Toronto, Ontario, Canada
M5E 1B3

Phone: 1-800-387-7164
Fax: 1-800-204-4140
E-mail: cservice@novalis-inc.com
www.novalis.ca

Library and Archives Canada Cataloguing in Publication
Pearson-Vasey, Gloria

    The road trip : life with autism / Gloria Pearson-Vasey and
J. Kevin Vasey.

Includes bibliographical references.
ISBN 2-89507-603-0

    1. Pearson-Vasey, Gloria, 1941–  2. Vasey, J. Kevin, 1969–
3. Parents of autistic children–Canada–Biography.  4. Autism-
Patients–Canada–Biography.  I. Vasey, J. Kevin, 1969–  II. Title.

RC553.A88P42 2005      616.85'882'0092      C2005-904709-7

Printed in Canada.

All rights reserved. No part of this publication may be reproduced, stored in a retrieval system, or transmitted in any form, or by any means, electronic, mechanical, photocopying, recording, or otherwise, without the written permission of the publisher.
We acknowledge the financial support of the Government of Canada through the Book Publishing Industry Development Program (BPIDP) for our publishing activities.

5 4 3 2 1        09 08 07 06 05

*Dedication*

*For those who journeyed with us,
helped us read the maps,
locate the roads,
and anticipate the destination.*

# Contents

Preface ..................................................................9
Introduction ........................................................11
1   Communication ............................................13
2   Community ...................................................36
3   Adjusting ......................................................52
4   Addiction ......................................................66
5   Resources ......................................................88
6   Relationships ................................................99
7   Hope and Dreams ........................................117
8   Limitations ..................................................130
9   Pioneers and Pilgrims ...................................149
10  The Quest for Meaning ................................163
11  Going Home ................................................177
12  The Advocates .............................................193
13  Confronting Rejection and Loneliness .........203
14  Pilgrims' Process ..........................................215
As Far as I Can Tell ..............................................228
Notes ...................................................................233

# Preface

*The Road Trip* did not begin as a pilgrimage – at least on paper. It was meant to be the documentation of a 1992 vacation tour of Atlantic Canada by my son Kevin, who has autism, when he was 23, and us, his parents. It originated as a collection of conversations transcribed first from a Sharpe Memo Writer, then an early digital communicator and, later, portable voiced computers.

The conversations spoke to the awakening of Kevin's communication skills. Documenting this transformation was a rejuvenating experience for my husband and me as we discovered our son's exceptional intelligence and had the privilege of seeing the world through his eyes. Because of Kevin's candour, we were allowed to glimpse the soul of a boy-man, at once innocent and wise, sometimes sophisticated, and often touchingly naive.

The documentation was, moreover, a journal of Kevin's ongoing struggle with addictions to solvent sniffing, cigarette-butt eating, and coffee "stealing." He expressed the hope that others with disabilities would benefit from his writings, be seen in an enlightened way, and thus be afforded respect and dignity.

This was Kevin's book and we were content that it stood on its own. But our editor wanted more. Where were the voices of Kevin's father and brothers? What was the story behind *The Road Trip*? Where are we today? How does Franciscan spirituality – in which my life is steeped – play into all of this? What of Kevin's own spirituality?

Initially I resisted, fearing it would no longer be Kevin's book. But as the manuscript evolved, I realized that it was becoming his book more than ever. The voices of Kevin's family, our shared history, our relationships with God and others – all of this makes Kevin who he is. Thus *The Road Trip* became the story of a pilgrimage. And so I thank editor Kevin Burns for creative nudging.

I am grateful also to my husband, Jim, and to our sons James, Christopher and Joel for their honest sharing of memories and convictions. I commend the individuals, management, staff and board members – past and present – of the St. Francis Advocates for their loving service to each other.

Numerous people and institutions deserve our family's gratitude. Five from the early, darker years warrant special mention: psychologist Irene Needham; physician Doug MacKinlay; therapists Elizabeth Berry and Diana Wilson Wright; and psychiatrist Dr. Abram Hoffer. I also thank the Integra Foundation for stepping in just in time, and our families for their eternal love and support.

The names of some people, places and institutions in this book have been changed to disguise their identity. Others have not, for they remain part of our lives.

*Gloria Pearson-Vasey*

*May 1, 2005*

# Introduction

This is the story of a journey. As in all journeys, there are maps to guide, roads to follow, and a destination to attain. Ideally, the maps allow ample opportunities for creativity, the roads are enticingly varied, and the destination is flavoured with mystery.

The journey threads its way through several dimensions. In one dimension, it is the account of a family trip to Nova Scotia. It is not the first such trip for this family, nor will it be the last. But there is something different and exciting this time: the journal is being logged by my son Kevin, a young man who has autism. He has expressed the hope that he might become a writer, tell others his story, and thereby enrich the lives of those who are similarly afflicted.

Kevin is travelling with us, his parents. His brothers, now grown, have made independent lives for themselves. Kevin has guarded dreams for his own future, a future that is compromised and complicated by his condition. He is also hoping that in Nova Scotia, birthplace of his adored maternal grandmother, he will find something of himself, something to inspire and motivate. For Kevin, the maps are hard to follow, the roads are often closed, and the destination is flavoured with uncertainty.

In another dimension, we travel back in time, and then ahead, along one family's personal journey. Like many young families, ours had set out with confidence. Barely aware of any need for maps, we savoured the variety proffered by the roadways, and anticipated the promise of the destination. But then we wandered into a dark and frightening place. The maps were riddles, the roads abruptly merged into a maze, and the destination was hidden from view.

Finally, we explore the journey in its spiritual dimension, a pilgrimage winding its way along the tortuous paths of life. In this dimension, there is always opportunity for creativity and discovery, even though the maps have been charted by those who have gone before. The roads are travelled with family and friends, mentors and seekers, sinners and saints. The destination is flavoured with the magnetic mystery of God.

And so we step into the first dimension, the one recorded in Kevin's journal in the summer of 1992, when he was 23 years old.

# 1

# Communication

**From Kevin's journal: The day before the trip**

"Kevin, I wasn't expecting you until tomorrow," I say. It is July 16, 1992, the evening before our trip to Nova Scotia is to begin. A counsellor from St. Francis House has dropped off our son, Kevin, vacation gear in tow, at our home.

"As far as I can tell, this is the day I'm to be here," he is quick to type. Kevin had been preoccupied with two things for several months: writing "a book about my life," and accompanying us to Nova Scotia, an experience he refers to as "the trip to the east." So we have decided to combine the two and create a journal of the adventure.

"When do you think we're leaving on our holiday?" I ask.

"Tomorrow."

Well, at least we're on track there.

I comment that he has two very large bags, and he explains that it's "because we're going on a long trip and that requires a lot of belongings."

It's wonderful to be able to carry on a conversation with our son after more than 20 communication-deprived years. I ask Kevin if he knows why Jim, his dad, is chuckling. "Because he likes to hear me talk," he replies. How very true!

"Dad should pack the car now," he urges, "because we're leaving tomorrow and he should leave early."

"But I have to work tomorrow," I remind him.

"As soon as you get home, we'll be waiting."

Is he trying to reassure himself or me?

Jim and I ask him about his most recent session with his addiction counsellor. "Did the counsellor say anything about coffee?"

"Yes. She said I could have real coffee two or three times a day, and drink juice the rest of the time. That seems okay. I'm not to eat [cigarette] butts at all."

"I agree with that, don't you?"

"Yes," replies Kevin. "That's not a bad idea."

"What about the pipe tobacco?" We have purchased a tin of pleasant-smelling pipe tobacco as an alternative to his ingesting used butts off the street. We hope it will be a lesser health hazard should Kevin have an overwhelming need for nicotine. Kevin seems unenthusiastic.

"If I want it," he types.

"Do you want some now?"

"Yes. But not yet."

"Do you think you can stop eating butts?"

"Yes, I will try."

Later I ask Kevin how he is. It's delightful to have him reply, "Excited. I can't wait until tomorrow."

"What are those sores on your leg?"

"I'm not sure, but I think it's a rash caused by solvent."

"Did you get into some solvent?" Along with his penchant for eating cigarette butts and stealing coffee, Kevin has long been addicted to solvent sniffing. Although much improved, he will still surreptitiously seek out various solvents.

"Yes, I rubbed paint remover on my clothes at SFH."

"Did anyone know about it at St. Francis House?"

"Yes, it was washed off by Norm."

Sometime later, Jim informs Kevin that we would not be going to Newfoundland this trip because we have been unable to get ferry reservations. "We'll go another time," he promises.

"I'm disappointed, because everybody thinks I'm going to Newfoundland," says Kevin.

"We still have lots to do with seeing Nova Scotia and Cape Breton," I remind him.

"That sounds fine. We will have as much fun. I'm glad we will see the relatives' places and graves. Nova Scotia and Cape Breton will be great."

"So are you happy?" I ask.

"Yes, I'm very happy. Are you happy I'm going with you?"

"I certainly am!"

"I was hoping you would say that."

My poor darling. He needs so much reassurance. And now I have a surprise for Kevin. Will he know what it is? "Look what I found in the attic, Kevin. Do you remember it?"

"Yes, it was my favourite Jay Jay. It talked and I pretended I was talking." Jay Jay is a toy figure modelled on a popular sitcom of the 1970s. It had a voice box activated by a pull string.

"It was the only gift you ever paid attention to," I comment. "You dragged it around all the time."

"Yes, I really enjoyed it. I want to take it with me to the east."

"Poor Jay Jay has lost his voice," I caution.

"Now Jay Jay can't talk but I can, and that's what counts."

"Yes. That's a pleasant irony," I say. "Why do you want to take it on holidays with you?"

"Because it's a possession of mine and a pleasant memory of my childhood."

I again address the matter of his baggage. "Kevin, I think you have too many things packed. You don't need towels or so many shoes. How be you just take one bag?"

But Kevin is adamant.

"No, I like to bring lots of things for our trip, and I even want the towels and the three pairs of shoes."

We watch television before going to bed. "Look, Kevin," I say. "*The Miracle Worker* is on TV. It's the story of Helen Keller, who was both blind and deaf."

"How could she understand anything?" he asks.

"At first she couldn't. But her teacher was very patient and taught her sign language."

"How could she see the signs?"

"She learned to feel them on her hand."

"That's wonderful. What is an asylum?" The word "asylum" has just been used on television, and Kevin has a way of running one thought into another on his memo writer. A speech pathologist recently told me that people who are dependent on assisted communication methods tend to do this. Whenever they get a chance to express their thoughts, she explained, they try to exchange as much information as possible.

"It's an institution," I reply to Kevin's question. "Helen's parents thought they would have to put her in one, because they would not be able to handle her as she got older."

"That would be terrible."

"But they hired Anne Sullivan to teach her, and she was able to live a mostly normal life."

"What could she do?"

"She wrote books, and encouraged other people to live enjoyable, productive lives whether they had handicaps or not."

"I would like to read about her."

"We'll get a book."

"So, where will we find one?"

"In a bookstore. Possibly on our holidays."

## Looking back: The family dimension

Kevin was born in the early summer of 1969, a seemingly normal, healthy baby. His first two years were a delight to us. He was happy and alert, and crossed all the appropriate milestones with flying colours. At twelve months, he had a ten-word vocabulary, and by eighteen months, he was reciting nursery rhymes and saying short sentences. Our family doctor and a pediatrician assured us that his chronic diarrhea and nasal discharge were no cause for worry, as he was obviously well nourished and healthy looking.

In the spring before his second birthday, he began to spend hours swinging on our backyard swing while singing "Baa, baa, black sheep," over and over and over. Unfortunately, we did not recognize this for the omen it was, but congratulated ourselves on our exceptionally "good" child. Within two months, we were jolted out of our complacency by a new, wild, screaming, destructive Kevin with whom we could do nothing. He reminded me of some frustrated stroke victims I had nursed: suddenly unable to express their simplest needs, or even understand much of what was said to them.

Now began a family trek through a never-never land of despair amid few short-lived hopes. Doctors, psychologists and clinic personnel shook their heads in bafflement. Endless tests and numerous visits to specialists of every discipline yielded no answers.

We registered Kevin at the local Children's Treatment Centre. The psychology of the sixties and early seventies stressed that *love* could cure all ills. This implied, of course, that most illness, and certainly all developmental setbacks, were caused by an *absence* of love. Kevin presumably would receive this missing affection at the Treatment Centre two mornings a week.

In order to bring him to the Centre, I had first to supervise the dressing and breakfasting of Kevin and his two older brothers (James and Christopher), load all three little boys into the car, and drop my husband, Jim, at the school where he was principal. The children and I would then return home for half an hour. At 8:45, I would send James, the oldest boy, off to school. Kevin, Christopher and I would drive to the Centre for Kevin's nine o'clock therapy.

Chris and I would return home for a brief two hours, then we would return to the Centre for Kevin's 11:30 pickup.

When we arrived at the Centre, I would discuss Kevin's morning with the staff. Kevin would be either riding obsessively on a rocking horse, or being held in a worker's arms upon a rocking chair in constant motion. College students, earning credits towards their Early Childhood Education diploma, would point out to me that Kevin needed lots of *love*. The director occasionally questioned me on my ability to cope with motherhood, and suggested that perhaps Jim was too busy for his sons.

Drained by suppressed angst and anger, I would rush home with the two younger boys, greet James, who was returning from his morning at school, and prepare lunch. James would return to school for the afternoon. This scenario varied somewhat with the seasons, being considerably more complicated by winter's snowsuits, mitts, scarves and boots. In the afternoons, I taught piano and theory from my home studio so I could be near my children and their sitter. On weekends, with Jim at home, I was on call in the operating room and emergency room departments of a local hospital in order to maintain my nursing skills.

During this time, preschoolers in our neighbourhood began participating in a co-op nursery school. My recollection of this period is rather hazy, but I know that Chris, Kevin and I were involved one or two mornings a week. Here, at least, I was with friends. When Christopher was four, he began attending Junior Kindergarten. Kevin continued to go to the Treatment Centre two or three mornings a week.

By Christmas of 1972, James was eight years old, Christopher was five and Kevin was three-and-a-half. Despite Kevin's destructive, unpredictable behaviour, we struggled to maintain a productive lifestyle for our sons. There were piano and swimming lessons, soccer and skating, cubs and scouts. There were dogs and cats – sometimes several pets at a time. And after school there were tutors for Kevin.

Then I found out I was pregnant. I kept this news a secret from family and friends for as long as possible. Jim and I both had family living less than three hours away, whom we visited regularly, but I did not want to ask for their help in any extensive way. Although they were concerned and supportive, and minded our children on occasion, I told myself that they were too busy with their own lives to have time for my problems. I was too anxious to admit, even to myself, how physically and emotionally drained I was.

Shortly after our fourth son, Joel, was born, Kevin, now age four, had a prolonged convulsion. Our family doctor hospitalized him for testing. Because an electroencephalogram showed "a left focal point," Kevin was sent to Children's Hospital in London, Ontario, not far from where we lived. There he was kept diapered in a covered crib. Because he was not free to use the bathroom and could not communicate his toileting needs, he was written up as "untrainable." I protested in vain that he was, in fact, reliably toilet trained.

A total of four weeks of in-hospital testing shed no light on his illness. In the last three decades, technical developments have provided a range of non-invasive neuroimaging. But in the early 1970s, a painful procedure known as an air encephalogram was still included in efforts to separate general medical conditions from mental disorders. This was the final diagnostic test performed on Kevin before he was discharged from hospital. Via a lumbar puncture, extracted spinal fluid is replaced with injected air, which rises to the brain of a patient held in an upright position. Because air can be seen in x-rays, intracranial abnormalities may thus be shown. Unfortunately, the process causes severe headache and frequently, as in Kevin's case, fever. A few days later, we brought home a frightened, confused and distrustful little boy. Now totally mute, Kevin was terrified of baths, shampoos and large buildings. His fear of medical personnel lasted for years.

Later in that fall of 1973, Kevin was accepted in a newly established Developmental Junior Kindergarten at St. Peter's School. As it happened, Jim was principal there, and for the following several years he would be seriously tested by the presence of his third-born son in his scholastic domain. Jim's later comments regarding this subject are a definite understatement. "I learned a great deal," he says. "The knowledge and the behavioural training we had helped me professionally. I think a good thing about me being principal of Kevin's school was that I was able to handle behavioural problems that might have been quite upsetting if he had been at another school." Over the years, Jim would receive awards for his creative, selfless work with disabled students, and for his persistence in defending their rights.

But back to 1973: at a Centre meeting in October, Jim and I were told that since no organic cause had been found for Kevin's withdrawal and lag in development, "we feel it is probably emotional withdrawal." Kevin would be placed in a play therapy program every Wednesday morning for an hour and a half. The school board mercifully brought Kevin by taxi to and from his play therapy sessions, leaving my mornings free for baby Joel and housekeeping.

In December of that year, Jim and I were again summoned to a Centre meeting. Ten people were in attendance, including Kevin's teacher from school. The Centre staff informed us that the play therapy program was not working out because Kevin interrupted the therapy of the other children. Moreover, it was their opinion that Kevin was "a very disturbed child who needs much more help"... perhaps institutionalization at the Browndale therapeutic homes.

The Director of the Centre implied that Kevin was suffering from emotional abuse. I recall even now how other staff seated around the table hardly dared look at me, and how one young therapist's hands trembled.

Stunned and angered by these unfair innuendos, I went home and phoned my friend Irene Needham, a retired psychologist with a background in nutrition and psychology. She assured me that Kevin was neither emotionally withdrawn nor very disturbed, as the Centre claimed. Her opinion was that Kevin had suffered brain damage from an undetected virus or an adverse reaction to vaccination. Or maybe it was a chemical imbalance or allergies.

"Look at your other little boys," she soothed me. "They're beautiful and well adjusted! Why should Kevin be disturbed?"

At Irene's urging, and desperate for answers, we took Kevin to an allergist and had the entire family tested for allergies. We altered our diet, and for a while, everyone in the family received allergy injections. At this point the Centre brought in psychiatrist Dr. Goldberg, from London, who diagnosed Kevin as having autism. In 1973, this was a grim prognosis. The following summer, we travelled to Saskatoon to receive counselling from Abram Hoffer, a psychiatrist specializing in biochemical therapy. We returned home armed with information on diet, megavitamin therapy and child management.

But over the years, Kevin's school achievement forms varied little. Kevin was "able to discriminate colour, shape, size, soft and loud sounds as well as rough and smooth objects." He could also assemble puzzles, insert small pegs into holes, and hum nursery rhymes. However, he pushed other children, ran out of the classroom, did not participate in circle time, and could not properly hold or control a crayon.

With the exception of a year in a regular Junior Kindergarten at a different school, Kevin remained in special education classes at St. Peter's. There were regular incidents of disruptive behaviours: "Kevin would not play with the other children... Kevin was eating banana peels from the garbage container... Kevin ran from the schoolyard, chasing dandelion fluff down the neighbourhood streets... Kevin was aggressive when asked to complete a task... Kevin tried to open the emergency door on the bus."

### Reading, writing and facilitation

The ability to read and write permeates our lives with richness, wonder, and the power that communication provides to social beings. Yet many lack the means of expressing their thoughts and yearnings. We were unacquainted with such concerns when we welcomed our firstborn into our lives in 1964.

Our children learned to read before they started school. I had read that if one teaches a child to read as a preschooler, there is then no chance of the child slipping through the cracks of the system and becoming illiterate. I took this warning very seriously. *My* children would not be slipping through the cracks.

It required more patience and persistence to teach Kevin, who had little speech and extremely unpredictable behaviour. We began each lesson tracing sandpaper alphabet letters while saying the letter's sound. Kevin then carried letters and flash cards to me as I asked for them. I would have several of these lined up on an easel, and Kevin would have to select the correct one. For each accurate response, Kevin would get a raisin. We went through a lot of raisins. We also used the assistance of teenage tutors.

As it turned out, it was fortunate that our sons were studying phonics at home at a time when it was not being stressed in the schools. Dr. Temple Grandin, who calls herself a recovered autistic and is an internationally recognized expert on animal behaviour, thanks her mother for teaching her phonics. "I would never have learned to read by the method that requires memorization of hundreds of words," she notes. "Old-fashioned phonics enabled me to learn reading. After I laboriously learned all the sounds, I was able to sound out words. Learning less than 100 sounds is easier than attempting to remember thousands of incomprehensible groups of symbols."[1]

Unlike Temple Grandin, Kevin's eclectic limitations do not permit him to function at her level of independence. Moreover, because he is mute, has a peculiar gait, and is given to odd, compulsive behaviours, people who don't know him well might overlook his intelligence and wit.

Autism describes a complex collection of neuro-biological disorders in which messages sent to the brain through the senses are not accurately processed and interpreted. Recently, researchers have found evidence pointing to chronic brain inflammation caused by immune system activity, beginning perhaps in the womb, and continuing throughout the life of a person with autism.

Like snowflakes, persons with this enigmatic condition are unique, and like all humans, have varying capabilities and difficulties. Especially frustrating to people with autism and to their associates, however, are the challenges surrounding communication. These include no speech, repetitive speech, and impaired conversational skills.

Although teachers creatively wrote encouraging statements about his academic progress year after year, Kevin did not advance beyond tracing or copying letters and numbers. He had, however, learned some sign vocabulary. Soon I no longer bothered to point out to teachers my belief that Kevin could read. In fact, my own certainty was fading.

Some years later, when Kevin was attending a residential school in Toronto, I was inspired to visit David Eastham in Ottawa. David was a young man with autism who communicated through typing. In meeting with David, his mother, Margaret, and his teacher, I became convinced that a new avenue had opened for Kevin. Like Kevin, David had been painstakingly taught to read by his mother using sandpaper letters and word cards. But David was communicating intelligently, and even writing poetry! At the time of my visit in the mid-1980s, he required only the touch of a pointer at his shoulder in order to type. (And before his early death by drowning, David had graduated to needing no assistance at all.)

Margaret Eastham explained to me that the reason David needed assistance to type was because he was apraxic. Apraxia is an impairment of learned movement that cannot be explained by deficits in language comprehension or motor function. The person is unable to convert clearly understood commands into movements, such as typing or turning off a light switch. Sometimes the person describes himself as being "stuck." Until then, I had never thought of Kevin as being apraxic, but it made uncanny sense, and explained many things.

Years earlier, when I had told doctors that Kevin seemed to have had a stroke, I was close but not right. A typical stroke patient has aphasia, not apraxia, and may neither understand language nor communicate meaningfully by any method. According to two researchers, "Aphasia should be diagnosed only when there are deficits in the formal aspects of language such as naming, word choice, comprehension, spelling or syntax."[2]

I asked David what I should do for Kevin, and he replied through his typing, "Teach him to read."

"He does read," I said, "but nobody believes me."

"Teach him to type," added David.

One of Kevin's residence counsellors had accompanied me to Ottawa, and she was as excited as I was by our new-found knowledge. With Shari assisting Kevin at school, and me working with him whenever we brought him home, Kevin's typing skills increased steadily. One day, however, I received a tearful phone call from Shari. The North York School Board had told her she had to stop the typing program immediately. They did not believe that Kevin was capable of communication at the level he was demonstrating, and accused Shari of typing for him, rather than merely providing support. When the typing program stopped, Kevin withdrew again into his world of silence, and became increasingly morose.

In 1987, Kevin returned home. Not long afterwards, information began to circulate concerning a "new" method whereby some people with cerebral palsy, autism and Down syndrome were able to type with hand-over-hand support. In the 1970s, Rosemary Crossley and her colleagues at The Dignity through Education and Language Communication Centre in Melbourne, Australia, had been able to facilitate with twelve children suffering from severe cerebral palsy.

Douglas Biklen, a sociologist and professor at Syracuse University in New York, observed Crossley in 1989. Biklen was amazed at the level of communication in Crossley's classroom.

> In light of the natural language produced by Crossley's students through typing, we are compelled to search for an alternative explanation for their mutism and unusual speech. The obvious interpretation is that they have a neurologically based problem of expression. In other words, their difficulty with communication appears to be one of praxis rather than cognition... This interpretation also presumes that while there may be peculiarities in vision and learning, such as involuntary attention to light or acute sensitivity to certain sounds, these do not necessarily reflect or create cognitive problems.[3]

What Margaret Eastham had discovered earlier in Ottawa was now being celebrated in Australia and the United States. Facilitated communication, or FC, as it was being called, had gained credibility, and Kevin was finally free to escape from what he has termed his "prison."[4]

Mastering facilitated communication is not without its trials. The entire process requires the careful training of facilitators and a great deal of patience on the part of the individual and all who support him or her.

It may take a long time for a facilitator and a user to bond and build up sufficient confidence to be able to work effectively together. Some users work very well with some facilitators and not at all with others. Some users will work only with a favourite teacher and not with a parent. On February 14, 1992, Kevin and I had the following conversation concerning his inability to facilitate with his teacher:

"Mrs. Buono is disappointed that you are not doing facilitated communication at school. What is the problem?"

"OENLTJFM KIM EAS IBMDYB." Kevin types a meaningless string of letters when he does not wish to talk or when he is uncertain of the answer.

"Yes, that is exactly the problem. You are writing nonsense. Why are you not talking to Mrs. Buono?"

"I don't know," he typed.

"You must have some idea."

"I always plan to talk but then I get scared."

"What are you scared of?"

"Of looking stupid."

"Writing nonsense doesn't look too bright."

"I know. I will try and do better."

"Is there something you would like to say to Mrs. Buono?"

"I'm sorry that I'm not always doing what you want me to do. I will do better this week," he typed. I had been hoping for a topic or situation he wished to discuss with his teacher, but Kevin apparently thinks I am looking for an apology or a promise of better things.

"One of the things Martha said today was that it's a good idea for people to work with many facilitators right from the start. That way they don't get used to just one person." Martha Leary is a speech pathologist and expert on autism who, working through the Geneva Centre, a provincially funded program, had supervised Kevin's progress for years. This afternoon, she had been a presenter on a Telemedicine in-service for Canadian hospitals. Several community professionals, including Kevin's teacher, had attended at the hospital site where I worked.

"Yes. I'm used to working with some people, and must learn to do it with other people."

"Mrs. Buono really wants to talk to you."

"I will certainly talk to her this week and say that I want to learn a new lesson."

"That will make her very happy."

"I think I would do better on my little computer." Kevin had a little Sharpe Organizer that he carried in his pocket on outings. It had no voice, but enabled him to order in restaurants, and communicate in other ways.

"Is that why you wanted to take it to school?"

"Yes," he said.

On March 3, 1992, we had a further conversation regarding communicating at school:

"Are you doing any better with facilitated communication at school yet?"

"No, I cannot seem to do it with the teacher."

"Are you still happy to go to school?"

"No, I would rather stay [at St. Francis House] and study with the staff."

"What should we do about school?"

"I want you to come to school and show the teachers how to facilitate with me," he said.

"What's happened with the Sharpe Organizer?" I asked. "Why did they send it back?"

"They think I'm stupid. They said Kevin can't do this work. His mother is lying."

"Did you hear them say that?" My stomach took a lurch. After all, I had reason to feel some trepidation. Prior to the introduction of Kevin's computer work at school, I had had an unforgettable, embarrassing experience where I felt my credibility, and indeed my sanity, were under scrutiny. I had been asked to show the classroom staff how to use facilitated communication. When I arrived at the school for the occasion, two superintendents and several teachers and assistants were waiting. One of the superintendents handed me his laptop and asked that I demonstrate the technique with Kevin. I was unfamiliar with the computer's ball cursor and Kevin was extremely anxious and agitated. We did not perform well.

"No, but I'm sure that's what they say behind my back," Kevin said now.

"I think they want very much to see you succeed. Somehow you must overcome this problem."

"You will have to please go to school every day," he pleaded.

How can one be certain that a user is communicating independently of the facilitator? There are some telltale clues. Facilitated communication is believable when the disabled user has his own distinct speech patterns and phrases. Kevin's language has a certain recognizable stiltedness and quaintness to it. As well, he often begins sentences with "as far as I can tell" or "perhaps."

Facilitated communication is believable when the user is focusing on the keyboard. It defies belief when a user is looking at the ceiling or twirling and spinning while looking in the opposite direction of the keyboard. Having said that, there is an issue of peripheral vision with autistic people. Kevin often looks at things from the side. He likes to watch television from the doorway of a room while standing sideways. When riding in a car, he often watches the passing scenery with his head facing frontward. Nonetheless, challenged users should be coached to pay attention to their work in order to improve both their accuracy and their image.

Facilitated communication is believable when the user is able to show signs of fading from the need of facilitating. Biklen refers to several students who are able to type independently – of these, all had been facilitating for more than three years.

When I facilitate with Kevin, I only need to touch his wrist with one or two fingers. But Kevin seems reluctant to take the final bold step to independence. We have been working on fading for some time, but the lighter my touch, the slower Kevin types. He says he "gets energy" from the facilitator.

It is possible that facilitated communication may not work for all autistic people. But for Kevin and many fortunate others, it has opened a window of opportunity onto the wider world.

Now Kevin can tell us what he likes about travel: "Seeing woods and streams and wilderness. Driving and looking at scenery and visiting museums and graveyards." He can explain the effects of his coffee addiction: "I feel happy and calm. I like to have more and more because it makes me feel happy. Too much makes me feel nervous and agitated. But none makes me feel nauseated and gives me a headache. Decaffeinated is worse than having none. I hate it and I would rather have juice."

Kevin's life has been further enriched by his new-found ability to communicate with brothers James, Christopher and Joel and their families. Although Kevin retains many of his unusual behaviours and social inadequacies, these continue to decrease. He now lives with two other young men in a small-town neighbourhood where all three receive minimal supervision and assistance from a single staff person on each shift.

Communicating with Kevin has taught us to question many commonly held beliefs about autism. For instance, contrary to textbook teaching, Kevin does seem to understand abstract concepts, metaphors, jokes, common sayings and idioms. This, however, makes it all the more challenging to make sense of his inappropriate social behaviours or his difficulties in sometimes following simple instructions.

In April 1992, when Kevin had been using FC only for a few months, his father had the following conversation with him at a Toronto hotel:

Jim: "I'm going to an ASO [Autism Society Ontario] meeting, and I'd like to give the people at the conference some of your insights. What should I tell them?"

Kevin: "Not being able to communicate is like being in a prison. It was not as bad when I was little because I was at home and my family had a way of knowing what I wanted. We used sign language."

Jim: "Is it frustrating being autistic?"

Kevin: "Yes, it is, and I get angry."

Jim: "What was difficult about school?"

Kevin: "I couldn't communicate my feelings to my classmates and teachers."

Jim: "How does facilitated communication work?"

Kevin: "I cannot talk and the computer tells me what to say. It helps me think because the letters are in my mind."

[Jim and I take this explanation in stride. It is just one more glimpse into our son's beautiful, kaleidoscopic mind.]

Jim: "What makes a good facilitator?"

Kevin: "They always hold my arm softly. It seems to steady my muscles and somehow almost seems to help me find the keys."

Jim: "When I tell people how important this is to you, other autistic people and their teachers and families will learn facilitated communication."

Kevin: "I hope so."

Jim: "What message would you like me to give people about facilitated communication?"

Kevin: "That it has certainly changed my life, because now I feel important and I can communicate like every other man who is intelligent. And I am treated differently than when people thought I was retarded."

Jim: "Can you go faster on the computer or on the organizer?"

Kevin: "I can mostly go fast when the keyboard is small. I mostly cannot get my hand to move faster."

Jim: "How does FC work?"

Kevin: "I'm sure there must be an explanation, but I don't understand it myself."

Jim: "What do you hope to do with your life?"

Kevin: "I hope to go to university, and I want to be a writer. I want to write my life story and tell people what it's like to be autistic."

Jim: "Is it sometimes difficult to tell your story?"

Kevin: "I hate to cry in front of anybody. I get emotional when I talk about all those years when I was unable to let anyone know I was in here."

Facilitated communication is both an ethical and a social justice issue. Every human being is created to interact with others of our species, and speech is critical to human interaction. Speech sets us above all other life on earth. The ability to communicate is our birthright. It is essential to our well-being. Jean Vanier has a story on this subject:

> A few years ago, I visited a large institution in Brazil It was about ten in the morning. I was surprised to find a room with about forty children with disabilities still in their beds and not one of them was crying. Children only cry out when they know and hope that someone will answer; they will not waste their energies if they are certain that nobody will hear. They will close up in despair; they have no hope.[5]

The Ontario Consultants on Religious Tolerance website agrees.

> We feel that there is a major ethical component to the current debate over FC.... If FC is proven to be a reliable technique for some people, then the current situation is unacceptable. FC is being banned and discouraged in many areas. To prevent access by disabled persons to an effective method of communication is analogous to locking an innocent person into solitary confinement and throwing away the key.
>
> If FC is a hoax, then the current situation is also unacceptable. FC is now being used in many locations. If the messages come totally from the facilitator and not from the client, then the autistic person is not really being heard. Time is taken away from other activities that might benefit the individual... It raises false hopes in parents and other caregivers.[6]

We who work with individuals using FC know it is not a hoax. One successful user is Andrew Bloomfield of Guelph, a young man we have known since he and Kevin attended Camp Towhee together in the mid-1970s. His twin sister, Victoria, who was also his best friend and only sibling, was killed in a car accident more than seven years ago, just after earning her Ph.D. Andrew's parents, Gerry and Elizabeth, have recently retired from teaching at the University of Guelph. They combine their lifelong commitment to research and writing with more than 30 years' involvement in the autism cause.

Elizabeth writes of her son,

> Andrew has his own home, directs his own life with the use of facilitated communicating, values friends, and is passionately interested in learning and in contributing to his community. He cares deeply about the environment and about spirituality. FC helps him to express himself reliably, though he also has a large sign vocabulary and can use PECS [language symbols]. Only with FC can his friends understand how "smart" (his word) he is, and how mature and realistic his insights are. For Andrew's FC to be accessible, he has to depend on others who believe in him. People who support Andrew in any way are interviewed and vetted by him. He

is very patient with their time of apprenticeship and learning from him. He has a nice way of saying, "I like this or that in XX, but I wonder if she is really happy...or really believes in me enough." After trying several times with some people, we have had to let some go on Andrew's say-so, with which we agree.[7]

Is it true that facilitated communication works only for a small number of people? Even if this *is* true, does it matter? It is crucially important that we do not eliminate people as potential FC users by our own biases. Supporters and critics of facilitated communication need to come to an agreement on a means of determining who can benefit from this important, life-altering method.

Communication is essential human contact. It is the pathway to understanding, bonding and love among beings created in the image and likeness of God. "The overall purpose of human communication is – or should be – reconciliation," writes psychologist M. Scott Peck. "It should ultimately serve to lower or remove the walls and barriers of misunderstanding that unduly separate us human beings one from another."[8]

Communication, of all things, should not be a wall separating those of us who love and nurture individuals who cannot speak for themselves or by themselves. Communication is a God-given gift and a critical necessity in human functioning.

**Spiritual journey**

Among my earliest vivid memories of childhood are train journeys to and from Nova Scotia with my mother. It is wartime and the trains are crowded with soldiers. There is noise and bustle everywhere, and I must hold tightly to my mother's hand as we run for the train. But she and I are happy and excited. We are travelling to see Daddy, who is posted at Halifax with the Canadian Navy, and to stay with Mommy's family on Cape Breton Island. My mother is going home, and so, by association, am I.

When we arrive in Nova Scotia, my mother is greeted by relatives joyfully crying, "Jesus, Mary and Joseph – it's Edie!" or "Thanks be to God, you're here!" It seems strange that what could pass for swearing in Ontario is a loving greeting here. There are exuberant hugs and kisses from Grandpa, Nana, aunts and uncles. Grandpa's mother, my great-grandmother, is working in her garden. She welcomes us into her house and gives me a very spicy gingersnap. I eat it to be polite. There are adventures to share over every hill with my free-spirited cousins.

After the war, regular holiday trips to Nova Scotia continued. But these became car trips with both of my parents and, over time, with brothers and sisters. Interestingly, the details of these later trips are not as sharply focused in my memory as are the trains of war. The imagery of train travel – scenery speeding by, wheels clicking rhythmically over tracks, the haunting whistle (is it calling or warning?), uniformed soldiers moving about, sleeper berths and curtained aisles – remains vivid to this day.

Being able to vacation in the Maritimes as a child provided me with a colourful, cultural contrast to my everyday life in Ontario. My Ontario kin were fewer in number, Protestant, and more reserved. It was a time when distrust and misunderstandings ran deep between Protestants and Catholics, a situation that I found confusing and disturbing. My father had converted to Catholicism while overseas during World War II. By then, his Orangeman father was dead and Dad no longer had to fear his wrath. We tended to play down religious talk within our extended family, although tensions did arise from time to time.

I adored my grandmother with whom we lived for several years in Leamington, Ontario. She answered my endless questions, told me stories of her childhood, read to me on demand, and took me shopping with her. Sometimes I would accompany her to Evening Service at the Anglican Church. As I got older, I was discouraged from doing this. I have no recollection of how this happened, whether it was gradual or abrupt. In hindsight, it makes me sad, as it must have made Grandma at the time.

Along with my memories of train travel in Nova Scotia, I have memory bites of lazy summer days in Leamington. On one such hot day in July, I am standing on our porch with my mother. It's the "Glorious Twelfth" – the day of the Orangemen's Parade. Across the street, a middle-aged neighbour rushes down her front steps, waving and shouting enthusiastically at passing cars bearing orange streamers. She knows, of course, that we are Catholic. My mother mutters as she retreats into our house in disgust. Later, though, she allows me to join a small crowd assembled on the corner a block from our house, one of several groups lining the parade route. As we restlessly stand there, we listen intently for the beat of drum, the stomp of feet, the clop of horses' hooves, and the roar of engines that herald the approach of the Orange Parade as it winds its triumphant way through the streets of town.

Children standing with me at the curb slyly ask if I know that the parade celebrates how the Protestants beat the Catholics. *Yes*, I think, and I am also aware that my own grandfather proudly participated in it during his lifetime. Should I feel shame? Should I feel pride? It's most unsettling. I say nothing, and decide to feign nonchalance. I have already learned the art of the stiff upper lip from my family, but I am too young yet to recognize or embrace the theology of suffering to which I am being gradually introduced.

Travelling to the Maritimes still stirs my heart. I feel the subtle but unmistakable pull of my ancestry calling me. In my memories, the Maritimes is a place of beautiful scenery, joyful welcome and carefree exploration. Wonderful things can happen here, *saints be praised* and *thanks be to God!* And so, as Jim, Kevin and I travel eastward in the summer of 1992, Nova Scotia beckons with both memory and promise.

People ask me how I survived the terrible years of coming to terms with Kevin's autism. I know now that it was God, present since my infancy, close even at times when I had stopped seeking God, who supported me. In the journey of life, we process our hurts and they become part of who we are. It is up to each of us to make them an enriching, useful part. Unknowingly, I had been absorbing a theology of suffering all along. It would be another ten years before I would become a Secular Franciscan, and study how Francis of Assisi had acquired the grace to find joy in suffering.

Early on in Kevin's illness, I behaved like the child I had been at the Orange Parade, feigning nonchalance. Preoccupied with concealing my hurt and fear, I played out a public role of serenity and competence. But this was not the Glorious Twelfth, and I couldn't run home to Mother while the horses, vehicles and marching bands faded off into the distance. Instead, it was I who had become a mother to little boys who looked to me for permission to watch the parade. Blessedly, parents are able to play their roles even while they're learning their lines.

In reality, I was terrified that Kevin could somehow be taken from me by misguided professionals. I was furious that the very people who should be helping me had become my enemies. I became suspicious even of family and friends, imagining that they thought we should take the easy way out and send Kevin away.

I agonized that I could be doing more to free Kevin from the condition that threatened to destroy his life. Surely there was an answer somewhere. I worried that my other sons were receiving half-hearted care from an emotionally absent mother. I bartered and bargained with God, and God was silent. My life had become a wasteland. It was difficult to see any beauty in such a place.

Kathleen Norris observes that the basic principle of desert survival is not only to "know where you are but to learn to love what you find there."[9] It took me a while to figure out where I was, and longer still to learn to love the circumstances in which I found myself.

# 2

# Community

**From Kevin's journal: Days 1 to 4**

Jim, Kevin and I set out in our car early the next morning. As we prepare to leave, Kevin is anxious and agitated. "Be sure to bring Jay Jay and my computer on our trip to the east," he types, then adds, "I'm angry Joel is not coming. I like being with him."

"Joel has to work. You know that."

"Yes. But it will not be the same."

"The three of us will still have fun."

"That will have to do."

The following day we cross into Quebec, and on the third day arrive in the Gaspé. As we travel, we listen to French audiotapes to brush up on our rusty high-school French. Finally Kevin types, "I'm tired of hearing that French tape."

"We want to be able to ask for things so that the French-speaking people know what we want," I explain.

"I didn't know that," Kevin acknowledges.

"Has the trip been nice so far?"

"Yes, it's been very interesting. I'm so happy to be with you and Dad. It's wonderful to travel and I hope we can do this every summer."

Along the way we discuss many things. I ask Kevin why he seems not to look at things directly. "I'm looking out of my peripheral vision," he replies promptly.

"What do you know about peripheral vision?" I ask.

"It's something I've known for a long time," he says.

As we seat ourselves in a restaurant, Kevin observes, "They're speaking in French."

"It would be nice if *we* could speak French," I sigh.

"Yes, that would make it easier to order our food," notes Kevin.

People have often commented that Kevin has a talent for overhearing conversations. This trip is no exception. "What did you say to Dad?" he asks at one point. Jim and I are having what we think is a quiet conversation about someday going to Italy, France and some other places in Europe. "I hope you will always take me. I want to go to Europe and pay my own way. I will save all my money."

"Sometime we will go to Europe," says Jim.

"When might we go?" he persists.

"Probably in about five years." says Dad. "How would we get there?" The school principal in Jim delights in testing Kevin's general knowledge.

"We would fly or travel by ship," says Kevin.

"Why not by car?"

"The ocean would get in the way," types Kevin, adding, "That's a foolish question."

Soon we experience one of the challenging episodes that Kevin regularly throws our way. He eats a discarded cigarette butt and runs in front of a car. The unlikely excuse for this alarming behaviour is, "I thought we were going to Mass."

"Are you ready to settle down?" I ask.

"As far as I can tell, I am calm. I will definitely stop. About going to Europe, do you mean I can go? That's the main reason I would stop eating butts."

Later, as we eat at a sidewalk café, Jim asks Kevin, "Do you think these umbrellas would be nice at home?"

"They're very nice for a café but they shouldn't have beer commercials for a house."

"What do you think of the food here?" I ask.

"Excellent," says the young connoisseur. Then he adds, "Perhaps we should go to a church and say a prayer for a happy trip. Perhaps then you and Dad could go to Mass alone."

"What is your problem with Mass?"

"Too crowded and noisy and smelly, and as far as I can tell we don't need to go there to talk to God."

What Kevin says here is in keeping with the hyper (or hypo) sensory symptoms associated with autism.

"We need to go to church to receive Jesus," I answer.

"I could receive Jesus from you if you brought communion to me."

"You need permission from the priest to do that."

"You did it before."

"Yes, with permission."

"Communion is important but I still don't like Mass."

"We expect mature behaviour from you, Kevin."

"I will try. Perhaps we could go once."

On July 20, we visit a shrimp factory on the Gaspé. All of us on tour are required to wear hairnets. Kevin promptly removes his.

"I feel silly wearing this hairnet," he types.

"Everyone visiting the shrimp factory has to wear one."

"I feel silly just the same. I don't enjoy looking like this. Do they kill them first?" Kevin is referring, of course, to the shrimp. In his usual fashion, he takes advantage of a typing moment to fit in more than one topic.

"I'm not sure if it's possible," I admit.

"That's cruel," declares Kevin. "They should figure out a way."

But Jim has a better explanation: "They die from the change in pressure coming out of the water."

"I'm glad they're dead before they're steamed," types Kevin. "Have you ever eaten shrimp?"

"Yes. It's delicious," I say.

"Let's stop at this seafood restaurant," suggests Jim.

It's a small, simple eatery, and Kevin has many astute observations. "This is nice. It was helpful that they spoke English. Why are we the only people here? It's taking a long time. Let's hope it's worth it. It has very nice food but the atmosphere is a bit strange. They have plastic cutlery and disposable dishes."

Later in the day we stop at a church. "We're going to visit this beautiful historic church," I inform Kevin.

"I like this church," he says. "It's perhaps Catholic." On entering a side chapel, he adds, "This is a good idea having a private chapel. It's much nicer than a noisy church. We should go to church on quiet days."

Our day is going nicely, but en route to Percé, Kevin begins to rock back and forth, shaking the car. We pull over, get out the Memo Writer and demand, "What are you so agitated about?"

"I want to understand about asylums. Why are they still there?"

"You're concerned about the institution we saw when we were leaving Gaspé," I comment. We had taken a little detour to check out an intriguing mansion, which proved to be a large residence facility, so I guess this has lingered in Kevin's mind. As for the word "asylum," has he remembered it from the Helen Keller movie we'd watched on the eve of our departure from home?

"Yes. I saw those people behind the windows," types an agitated Kevin.

I, too, had noticed people rocking to and fro through the glassed-in porches.

"There is not enough money for smaller homes," I try to explain. "Also, many of those people don't have families to care for them."

"That is terrible."

We try to reassure. "Things are gradually changing, and more and more handicapped people are staying in their own communities."

"I will write about those people so others know they are there." Through the process of communicating, Kevin has grown calm. Not only has he been able to express his fears and concerns, but he has come to believe in his own power to be a voice for others in society.

## Challenging the social norms

Kevin sees institutions or "asylums" as fearful places where individuals are deprived of freedom and separated from those they love. This was in fact the fate of many vulnerable people during the "asylum era for the feeble-minded" that flourished from 1860 to the 1960s.

But it is not my intent to discredit the place or usefulness of institutions. After all, institutional thinking is embedded in our culture. Today, on a widespread basis, we are seeing smaller businesses, schools, school boards, health-care centres and hospital boards swept up into large conglomerates. It is said that this is fiscally responsible and for the greater good.

And so it is not difficult to understand that people in decades past also saw value in doing things on a larger scale. "The asylums created a place for mental deficiency within the social order, and it was widely believed this place was both proper and beneficial, not only for society but also for those who were 'mentally deficient.'"[1]

This was also the time when Aboriginal children were separated from their families and sent away to residential schools. Canadian and American governments believed it would be to the children's (and the governments') advantage for Native children to become versed in European ways and the Christian faith. But the residential school system alienated children from their culture, their religion and their families without preparing them to fit into a different society. "Worst of all," writes First Nations author Harold Cardinal, "perhaps, the entire misconceived approach, the illogical (to the Indian children) disciplines enforced, the failure to relate the new education in any pragmatic way to their lives turned the child against education, prevented him from seeing or appreciating the benefits of a real education."[2]

Current beliefs do not favour routinely separating any children from their families. All children, including those with disabilities, belong in their home communities. As late as 1970, however, there still existed 20 asylums for the "feeble-minded" in Ontario, and 21 more in the rest of Canada. These numbers do not include institutions for the mentally ill, which before 1860 also housed "mental defectives."

But neither was the *pre*-asylum era ideal for disabled persons. "Some were cared for at home, others depended on charity, either on their own or in places such as houses of refuge or insane asylums, and still others undoubtedly ended up in prison. There was poor access to medical help, and, partly because of this, infant mortality was high and life expectancy short."[3]

Society changes its concept of appropriate terminology. People with developmental disabilities have been variously called "feeble-minded," "idiot," "mentally deficient," and "retarded," to name a few terms. The buildings that housed these people were given labels shocking to current thinking. For example, the Ontario Asylum for Idiots, situated on Lake Couchiching near Orillia, had an equally dismaying title earlier, when it was a branch of the Toronto Lunatic Asylum. Radford and Park report that "in 1906, Ontario was sufficiently concerned about the problem of feeble-mindedness to appoint an Inspector of the Feeble-minded, Dr. Helen MacMurchy, who held the post until 1919."[4]

In the late nineteenth and early twentieth centuries, Western society became convinced that poverty, prostitution and slums could be eliminated by controlling the reproduction of particular social groups. Known as eugenics, a process began in Britain where persons deemed "offenders" could be detained in asylums during their reproductive years on the grounds of low intelligence. In the United States, sterilization and custodial segregation were both implemented by 1927. Sterilization programs were established in Alberta in 1928, and in British Columbia in 1933. More than two thousand people were sterilized in Alberta alone before the law was repealed in 1971. Although Ontario officially relied on custodial segregation, it is considered "unlikely that the province remained free of eugenic sterilization procedures."[5]

It is true today, as always, that parents must advocate strenuously for their disabled children's rights and well-being. But from the 1940s through the 1970s, professionals in the behavioural sciences, being largely Freudian-trained, put parents with autistic children through hell. Books like Bruno Bettelheim's *Empty Fortress* fanned the flames of parent abuse by blaming autism on cold, negligent mothers. Some relief came in the 1970s, with the release of publications by Dr. Lorna Wing of England and American psychologist Dr. Bernard Rimland, both of whom had autistic children of their own. By that time, people with developmental disabilities were less likely to be admitted to "hospitals for the mentally retarded," as they were now called.

Psychiatrists and psychologists were gradually beginning to think of parents as partners in their children's therapies, rather than nuisances. However, many still believed that there were some whose needs could be met only in the safety of the asylum. "Family members who had placed their relatives in closed institutions were often worried by the prospect of having to provide unaccustomed care in their homes. Many others were concerned – with some justification as it turned out – that the savings from institutional closure would not be fully re-invested in community services."[6]

Thus, while some voices began to clamour for community-based care, families who had placed their relatives in institutions were resistant and fearful. One concern, as noted above, was that savings from institutional closures would not be transferred to provide replacement care in home communities.

To date, families with severely disabled children living at home are still waiting for the equivalency of funding assistance they would have received had their children been placed in institutional care. Instead, they struggle alone, with minimal help at best, to care for these family members. School and workshop placements provide relief. But during weekends, evenings, nights and holiday periods, they are mostly on their own. Many are physically exhausted, emotionally depleted, and imprisoned in their homes.

Where does a family turn today? No longer is there access to an institution to provide a long-term solution to the stress and strain. Instead, there is the end-of-the-rainbow promise of community resources. There are many caring professionals but a shortage of money to provide services. Both creativity and persistence are needed. Promising planning tools, such as Circles of Support and PATH: Planning Alternative Tomorrows with Hope, are becoming increasingly popular. Initially, trained facilitators work with the person with a disability, his or her family, and various friends, professionals and acquaintances to brainstorm about the individual's current lifestyle and personal vision for the future. Thereafter, a committed group meets on a regular basis to help the person pursue goals and seek opportunities for a meaningful and secure future.

It is now generally believed that persons with disabilities should be integrated into the mainstream of education and work. My husband, Jim, pointed out to me recently, "The Catholic separate schools of Ontario were better at this back when Kevin was in school, partly by happenstance. The public school boards had more money for separate buildings. Therefore, many municipalities had marvellously equipped schools for handicapped children – but they were segregated.

"Classes need sufficient numbers of teacher assistants to work with the many students of varying needs. There are fewer now," notes Jim, "than in Kevin's time. What is also needed is programming help. There is too much emphasis on testing and diagnosis, and not enough help or time for the development of a day-to-day progressive program."

Kevin's eldest brother, James, says,

> People with disabilities should be provided with the care that I [as a tax payer] would expect if I woke up one morning disabled [autistic]. I would of course expect adequate food, clothing and shelter, and I would expect every opportunity to learn to become a contributor to society. I would expect reasonable and qualified people to make reasonable and educated attempts at ensuring I learned as much as possible in a positive learning environment. Furthermore, I think

that we as Canadians now know that in order to provide a positive learning environment to persons with disabilities it will simply cost more than for the average student. There are accessibility issues, more one-on-one teaching required, and perhaps 24/7 care needed in some cases.

To this, Christopher adds,

I think that it is in society's best interests to find schools that focus on rigorous early education for people with disabilities. There are many people who learn to overcome their disabilities to make positive contributions to society. I realize that this type of education, requiring a low teacher-to-student ratio, can be expensive. However, it is short-sighted to reject this approach because of a high front-end cost. Society has a moral obligation to give people with developmental disabilities the best chance of a positive and good life. For those worried about cost, they need to consider the cost of supporting someone for life who might have otherwise become independent and self-sufficient had they had the proper early intervention.

This type of education is best provided in the regular school setting. It's a good life experience for students with disabilities and non-disabled students to interact with each other. I think that any temptation to set up "special" schools should be avoided. This can be a slippery slope leading to an out-of-sight, out-of-mind philosophy that was so prevalent in the past.

It depends on the disability [says Kevin's younger brother, Joel]. People with disabilities should have whatever resources are available to make them comfortable. I've always felt that social habits are more nurture than nature, so any child should be exposed to "normal" social settings as much as possible. Isolation or profiling should be kept to a minimum.

Families must continue to press for services and justice. It may be tedious, but this is the grace of community. We are created by God to live in community, and family is the basic unit. The needs of individuals are met when families and other advocates bring these needs to the community's conscience. I am very proud of Kevin's brothers and their spouses for their commitment to Kevin's and each other's well-being.

## The family as community

The family is a community wherein each person occupies a specific position and has a particular role. A healthy family respects the role of every member and celebrates each other's gifts. This respect and celebration extends, of course, to any member who is more vulnerable than the others.

It is also necessary to acknowledge and value differences. A baby soon comes to appreciate diversity. She notices differences, and is fascinated by them. Young children will happily point out characteristics of distinction. "Look, Daddy. That man has a brown face!" Rather than hastily dragging the child off in embarrassment, we might say something like, "Yes. He's very handsome." Similarly, when a child notices someone with a disability, we can respond with a positive comment while continuing nonchalantly on our way. We are all different in one way or another. We are all vulnerable to some degree.

When a family contains a vulnerable child, parents must make an ongoing effort to devote time, attention and love to their less vulnerable children as well. It is all too easy to become absorbed in the care of a child who is ill or has problems. Sometimes it may be necessary to remind professionals that we cannot neglect our other children, who are not in their program. They may then have alternate suggestions.

As part of the greater community, friends and relatives enrich our lives. In times of difficulty, we need them more than ever. Even when they have busy schedules of their own, family and friends can provide support and understanding. When extended families are separated by distance, it requires effort to stay in touch. But we should keep in mind that the opposite of kinship is isolation.

Although community sharing is reciprocal, even in the perfect community, it's easier to give than to receive. We are not good at asking for help. We are reluctant to admit that we need assistance.

We recoil from imagined pity while freely offering compassion to another.

And so we must work at community. We must dare to reach out to those in need. We must ourselves be brave enough to ask for help. "A group becomes community in somewhat the same way that a stone becomes a gem," writes M. Scott Peck, "– through a process of cutting and polishing."[7]

He adds, "The great enemy of community is exclusivity. Groups that exclude others because they are poor or doubters or divorced or sinners or of some different race or nationality are not communities; they are cliques – actually defensive bastions against community."[8]

A family in pain has a unique opportunity to *teach* community. Exposing our own vulnerability demands respect. Revealing our pain demands compassion. Demonstrating unconditional love for a disabled child insists on acceptance. Asking the community for aid creates the need for inclusion.

**Spiritual journey**

Many people relate that they have had a special God moment sometime in their lives. Although such a moment has been described in many ways, it is a mystical experience during which one feels completely embraced by the close, loving presence of God. Before I became aware that this was a universal experience, crossing cultural and faith systems, I believed that my own God moment was an extremely rare event.

It happened in the midst of my despair when Kevin was about five years old. I was alone in the living room of our house on a dark, rainy afternoon. The children were downstairs watching television in the den. It must have been a school holiday.

Weeping in anger and hopelessness, I raged at God. I can't imagine how you can be so cruel, heartless, and unfeeling! How can you inflict such a fate upon an innocent child? How can you ignore the suffering of a family? I trusted you and you're despicable! Why would anybody with a mind even believe that you exist?

In my misery, I demanded a sign proving God's existence, expecting nothing but oppressive silence. Suddenly, I felt myself wrapped in indescribable peacefulness and love. Warmth and visible sunlight brightened the room. There was no voice, no glowing presence, but I knew with certainty that I was embraced by Jesus. Later I would ask myself why I specifically believed that it was Jesus, especially when I had been hurling insults at the almighty God-of-aloofness. But I had the absolute conviction that God had come to me in the compassionate Jesus-person of the Trinity.

The experience faded, and I remember walking to the window to look for the sun. It was dark and sunless outside. Rain streaked against the windowpane. Yet an incredible peace and joy continued to envelop me. In the ensuing years, I have felt the presence of God, but never again in such a palpable way.

Skeptics have pointed out that experiences of God vary according to religious beliefs. A Jew reaches out to his Maker, the Holy One, blessed be He. A Muslim communicates with Allah. But this is hardly reason for doubting the existence of God. Rather, it is further proof of a God who relates to us personally, lovingly honouring our differences. Rabbi Hayim Donin relates that there are special times "when I want to cry out to the Supreme Being, to communicate with Him in a way that I can communicate with no one else. I cannot see Him, but He is real. He is there"![9]

What do we do with these special God moments? We turn them over in our minds and hearts for a while, and then we integrate them into the core of our ever-developing faith. Franciscan priest and author Richard Rohr says that God enters people's lives unexpectedly in order that we may acquire a sense of the sacred.

But he warns that seeking transcendental, emotional experiences can become a "cheap substitute for real faith…which means to believe and to know – without experience and without feelings. We might have to spend a whole lifetime walking in darkness, experiencing the little we've experienced in the light."[10]

How do we receive the gift of faith? How is it passed on to our children? God is revealed to us in all of creation, through scripture, and through tradition. Religion, the particular way we see God, is passed on from parent to child. In our case, we sent our children to Catholic schools. They accompanied us to Sunday liturgies. When Kevin types in his journal, "I could receive Jesus from you if you brought communion to me," his faith is a composite of grace, trust and experience.

Faith in God is especially important for the vulnerable and marginalized of the world. Blessedly, it is most accessible to them. We see this in developing countries, in ghettos and in prisons. Yet it is not the opiate of the masses, as Marx said. It is a gift of God, freely given, recognized most readily by the poor of heart. Unlike opium, it is life giving.

In 1983, when our youngest son was ten and his brothers in their teens, I joined a group studying the Rule and Life of Francis of Assisi. I was vaguely seeking a closer relationship with God amidst the chaos of my life. I was hoping, too, that I might attain some serenity and joy to pass along to my family. After all, was Francis not joyfully serene as he danced among animals, talked to birds, and kissed lepers?

I was to learn that Francis's appreciation for nature and lepers developed only after a radical change of lifestyle. Because his family belonged to the merchant class, Francis was raised to believe that a certain level of status, power and material comforts was his due. Following a bout of illness and time spent as a prisoner of war, Francis had a conversion experience during which the crucified Christ spoke to him in the crumbling church of San Damiano.

While meditating on the poor, broken body of Jesus, Francis became aware that the status, power and material comforts he had once worshipped had blinded him to his need for God. His affluent living, he realized, had been his god, a god demanding nurturing, expansion, defense and even war. Francis wept for the arrogant, selfish man he had been, and the God he had neglected.

So Francis became a disciple of Jesus, leaving everything behind in the manner of the first disciples. Others observed his new inner peace and joined him, wanting the same. The Little Brothers, as Francis now called them, worked among lepers, preached the Good News of Jesus far and wide, and begged for their food.

As his spirituality deepened, he became more attuned to seeing God in all of creation, and loving Christ in society's outcasts. Francis had learned that freedom is the fruit of simplicity. And that is why legends abound concerning Francis as a person of peace and joy. That is why he has become patron of ecology and protector of the earth's marginalized peoples.

Clare of Assisi, co-founder of the Franciscan tradition, was born into a family of nobility in 1193 when Francis was eleven years old. From an early age, she was prayerful and compassionate towards the poor. After his conversion, Francis visited Clare because of her notable holiness. Clare, for her part, responded to Francis's charismatic preaching by seeking his assistance to serve Christ as he did. Although she wished to live the lifestyle of the friars, Francis established her as abbess in the convent of San Damiano, which was more appropriate, and certainly safer, for women of that period.

Francis loved simplicity so much that he personalized it, calling it Lady Poverty. Similarly, Clare made the "privilege of poverty" the primary identity of her Poor Ladies. Francis "wanted to be identified with the lowest strata of society, which carried the negative connotations of dependency and legal incapacity. For Clare, poverty primarily meant identity with the poor Christ."[11] Clare described her vocation as a call to live in community in imitation of Christ.

She built unity among her Poor Ladies by their common commitment to the gospel and in their unity of mutual love. Clare's *Rule* states that the abbess is to "consult with all her sisters on whatever concerns the welfare and good of the monastery; for the Lord often reveals what is good to the lesser."[12]

In the earliest years of Franciscan development, lay people living with their families desired to live the spirit of Francis in their secular state. Francis encouraged them, and they became known as the Third Order Secular, now called Secular Franciscan Order. As with any religious order in the Church, a period of formation divided into inquiry (postulancy) and candidacy (novitiate) is required before one can be Professed into the Order.

When I became a Secular Franciscan postulant, I was not consciously seeking community. But community, I would come to realize, is a primary grace of Franciscanism. It is the means of living out the spirituality modelled by Francis and Clare. As we read in the Acts of the Apostles, Christian community has existed from the beginning of the Church.

> All who believed were together and had all things in common; they would sell their possessions and goods and distribute the proceeds to all, as any had need. Day by day, as they spent much time together in the temple, they broke bread at home and ate their food with glad and generous hearts, praising God and having the goodwill of all the people. (Acts 2:44-47)

I was pleased when Jim decided to become a Secular Franciscan, too. It's a blessing when a married couple can journey together spiritually. Jim says he joined the Order because of my faith, which prevailed "even when it was sorely tested." I am bemused that he would be thus affected by my wobbly faith, knowing me as he does. Jim also says that he has "never blamed God." This, too, is interesting in light of the fury that I have unleashed against God. Such is the strength of the family as community. We sustain each other as the situation warrants. We see the best in each other, we accept the faults and weakness that are there, and we model goodness for each other.

One of the highlights of our Franciscan journey has been the six years we served together on the Trillium Region Secular Franciscan Council. During that time, Jim, as Minister, and I, as Formation Director, had the privilege of receiving Franciscan hospitality as we visited local fraternities throughout Ontario. It was a time of spiritual growth for us as we met many inspiring people at regional and national planning sessions, workshops, conferences and retreats.

The Rule of the Secular Franciscan Order instructs us to devote ourselves "especially to careful reading of the gospel, going from gospel to life and life to the gospel."[13] In striving to live the gospel life, we model our lives on the ministry and teachings of Jesus Christ, following the examples of Francis and Clare. One could ponder this forever. It is so wonderful, so exciting, and so inspiring.

Clare and Francis based their spirituality on the life, death and resurrection of Jesus Christ. Through the Incarnation and Passion, God gave us a human Jesus with whom to journey. Through the Resurrection, God gave us a divine Jesus with whom to share eternity.

In Francis and Clare, God gives us saints to inspire and lead us along the way. "The pilgrim way is communal, and in the shared journey the I finds its true identity."[14] The lives of Clare and Francis echo the message of Jesus that we acquire unity of spirit, sympathy, love for one another, a tender heart, and a humble mind.

# 3

# Adjusting

**From Kevin's journal: Days 5 to 7**

*Day 5–July 21, 1992 – Percé*

"It should be a good day," types Kevin. "However, as far as I can tell, Dad is not in a good mood. What did Dad write? Was it about addictions?" Indeed, Kevin's addictive and obsessive behaviours *have* been taking a toll on our holiday atmosphere.

Jim: "I'm concerned that your mother is not getting the rest she needs on this holiday. All day long she's looking after you, and she gets upset when you keep eating butts. Then you're up during the night clapping, and she doesn't get the sleep she needs. I'm really fed up."

"I hope you're not planning to take me back and have a holiday without me," types Kevin.

Jim: "I'm seriously considering it."

"As far as I can tell, addictions are hard to control and are a sort of sickness. You should try to understand about this."

Jim: "I'm worried about your mother not having a relaxed holiday. She's too worried about you eating butts."

"As far as I can tell, she should stop worrying."

Jim: "Do you want us to ignore you when you eat butts, and let you poison yourself and die?"

"No, I don't want you to let me poison my body and die. Forget about worrying though, because that doesn't do any good. You should have a short holiday when I'm on the St. Francis House holiday." Kevin will be going on a holiday with his housemates later in the summer, and he is reminding us that this should provide us with respite.

"What made you think Dad was writing about you?" I ask.

"As far as I can tell, Dad was worrying about something, and I could feel that it was about me, and I was afraid he would take me back before he finished the long holiday, and I have been thinking about this trip to the east all year. It would be a terrible thing to do," Kevin types.

"We *want* to keep you with us."

"I know, and we should continue to enjoy ourselves."

Jim: "Another concern is that you're always running ahead of us instead of staying close to us."

"I will stay close to you from now on."

"Do you remember when you were here before, with your brothers?" I ask.

"We were just little boys. It makes me happy because I belong to a perhaps great family. I'm not sure I remember. Perhaps it will come back to me."

*July 23, 1992 — Moncton*

"As far as I can tell, it's a bit silly doing fighting and arguing," types a grumpy Kevin.

"I didn't realize we were," I say.

"I guess you have tried but it's hard to stop arguing."

"It seems that *you* are usually involved."

"No, you're arguing about other things, too. I guess you don't argue any more than other people, but why do they argue at all?"

Jim: "Perhaps you would rather go back to St. Francis House."

"What does Dad mean by that? He should know that I can't do that. Why is he annoying me? Dad should know that I try to be good. I want you to tell Dad I try. I should be able to feel secure and not always have to worry about you taking me back."

**Family values**

In comparing horror stories with other parents who raised autistic children in the sixties and seventies, I now realize that two important factors made us luckier than most. First, we had an empathetic family physician, Douglas MacKinlay, with whom I had worked in the hospital. Knowing me professionally, he had confidence in my mothering instincts. Thanks to his referrals, we were at liberty to consult with allergists and a biochemist psychiatrist at a time when both disciplines were controversial.

"No one knows much about autism. So if you're willing to experiment, I'm certainly not going to stand in your way," Doug assured me.

Second, Kevin was not an only child. Our other sons gave us confidence that we were on the right track as parents. They were healthy, well-adjusted boys, despite the extra demands placed upon them by having a brother with a serious disability.

"Siblings may experience various stresses in terms of embarrassment, increased chores, and less parental availability," note Lee and Gotlib in the *Handbook of Developmental Family Psychology and Psychopathology*. "However, living with an impaired sibling is not necessarily a harmful experience; indeed, it may even be associated with such positive effects in the sibling as greater maturity, supportiveness, and tolerance."[1]

> Certainly our own children's reflections on their childhood would bear this out.
> 
> Reflecting back to my childhood and youth [says James], my experiences were mixed. I thoroughly enjoyed travelling across North America as a family during the summers, trips that might not have occurred without having to seek out medical advice for Kevin. It brought our family (although somewhat reluctantly) closer together. On the other hand, simple outings during the rest of the year, such as going to a movie, or to church, for that matter, seemed much more

difficult than for other families. Kevin would often become agitated, loud and aggressive in public, and I think as soon as the opportunity arose for me to do things with my friends instead of with my family, I jumped at it.

As I grew older, I was often worried about what my peers and friends thought, especially girlfriends. I knew that they had a general understanding of the challenges my family encountered, yet I guess at some level I was concerned that it would scare them away from me eventually.

As a parent now, I realize that trying to devote time and energy to Chris, Joel and me must have been extremely difficult for our parents due to the constant care and attention Kevin required. I think that my childhood was as normal, as happy, and as nurturing as any of my friends' childhoods. Given the circumstances, that is a real credit to my parents.

Our second son, Chris, comments,

When I was young, I didn't have the impression that my family was much different from other families. Because Kevin and I are so close in age, I have always known him to be autistic and to display the behaviours that go along with that. As I grew older, there were responsibilities that were given to us, mainly focusing on watching Kevin when my parents were busy or away. I didn't perceive this to be much different than being in a family where large age gaps between children would require an older sibling to look after much younger children.

There are numerous cases where having a sibling with autism caused friction or was a source of embarrassment when dealing with people in the neighbourhood or at school. However, this was not the case within our family, and I believe our family life was relatively normal.

I'm often asked what life was like with a brother with autism, and my answer always seems to catch the inquirers off guard [says Joel]. I simply answer, "Kevin's my brother, just like Chris and Jim." I really have never had any what-if thoughts about life without Kevin. That being said, I've always felt my family life was pretty normal. Being the youngest probably made it easier for me. Never once have I asked someone, "How was your family life *without* a person with autism?" I guess I feel every family has its highs and lows, goods and bads. Our family is, and was, no different. I was pretty happy as a child.

Positive adjustment among family members relates more to resources within the family than to problems around the autistic child. According to Lee and Gotlib, "Thus, perceptions of the adequacy of social support, family cohesiveness and expressiveness all seem to be more promising predictors of favourable family functioning than is severity of the child's disorder."[2]

Psychiatrist Peter Szatmari of Chedoke-McMaster Hospitals says that the gift of persons with autism is that they see the world in a different way, and have "a very important capacity for seeing things in a special light. But they can't leave that different world, and that's the tragedy. The children suffer terribly, and their families suffer too."[3]

With autism being so poorly understood in those days, we did suffer. We endured stares and glares, and we expended a lot of energy seeking miracle cures. Looking back through the veils of time, I wish I could have had more fun with my precious little boys. I wish I had been less anxious and fearful, and not such a perfectionist.

Nonetheless, I do remember wonderful holidays of travel and camping across Canada and the United States. Because Jim was a school principal, he had entire summers off. Pulling a tent trailer, and with our car packed with boys, books, games, at least one dog, and sometimes a cat or two, we left our cares behind.

For weeks on end, there were no ringing phones and frantic schedules. No appointments with doctors, teachers, speech pathologists, dentists, psychiatrists, or play therapists. No soccer games, swimming lessons or music to practise. No homework or science fairs. No rushed mornings and exhausted evenings.

Just blissful drives through rolling country, lazy days of sun and sandcastles, relaxed evenings of marshmallow roasts and sleeping bags. "Contrary to expectations," say Lee and Gotlib, "the data with respect to marital adjustment indicate that parents of autistic children show levels of marital adjustment that are comparable to those demonstrated by happily married couples."[4]

As Jim says, "There is no doubt that having an autistic child greatly changes family life, yet I think we have done quite well. The fact that Kevin was the third one in the family took away the 'cold parent' blame that was laid on many parents, at least in our own eyes. That was important, because feeling we were normal parents gave us strength to carry on."

There were many challenges, such as Kevin's unexplainable outbursts in public, his running away, and his need to be tied at campsites. Yes, we actually resorted to tying Kevin in place, with a twelve-foot rope, while camping, and yes, we did endure derogatory comments from people passing by. But these same people had not been with us while alarmed park rangers and other searchers combed woods and trails for a missing boy. They had not been with us while police and neighbours scoured roads and railway tracks, fearfully calling the name of a lost child. Over time, we developed a maturing acceptance of Kevin's condition and adapted our lives accordingly.

"One of our difficulties, however, was a lack of social friendships," says Jim. "Since at least one of us had to stay home with Kevin, we didn't develop the kind of friends who golf together or invite each other over for barbecues. Our lives are still governed by Kevin's comings and goings, but I accept this as the way it is."

Knowing all I know today, would I manage my life differently? Undoubtedly, but I am suspicious it would not be as different as I imagine. Our natures seem largely pre-programmed. More and more, I look in the mirror and see my mother looking back, or I find myself doing and saying things she would do or say.

In raising our children, I believe I *might* try for less busyness and fewer activities. But how do parents know they don't have a potential concert pianist, violin prodigy, budding hockey great, developing golf pro, or promising ballerina?

Jim and I followed the parenting dictates of the times: Dr. Spock told us the parent must be in charge. Doman instructed us to teach our babies to read. Suzuki said we should use the infant's natural language-learning ability to learn the language of music. And so there was daily practicing and the nagging that goes with it. There were the stresses of recitals, festivals, and the driving to and from scouts, soccer, swimming, skating and, in high school, football. We have since decided that it is not the method used or the choices of family activities that matter. What really counts is loving attentiveness.

In fact, we were blessed with many good things: supportive families and friends, access to community resources, our own education and training, and trust in God. Along with all this, we had the good fortune of being able to participate in extended family leisure summer after restorative summer. As for Kevin, he was definitely helped by the many therapies he received, and shaped by developmental processes within his family. Slowly, he became calmer, more manageable and more attentive. His speech increased, and he developed a marvellous sense of humour, often manifested through his teasing of family members and our pets.

Looking back through the lens of time, if I could, I would post this memo in a prominent place in our home: Plan for tomorrow but live in the present. Cherish each day. Be kind and respectful, and expect the same. Give your cares over to God. Proceed with love, simple living, and common sense. These are the ingredients of serenity.

Then I would follow my heart. There would still have to be music, travelling and pets. Because Jim and I both love these, naturally we would want our children to experience these gifts of Creation. One of our sons, Joel, says he wishes we had exposed him to hockey. But we chose to be music parents instead of hockey parents. Both lifestyles make heavy demands on family time. We are content with our decisions. Our children became quite accomplished musicians and developed a lifelong appreciation for music. They were seasoned travellers and became knowledgeable about life throughout Canada and the United States. They grew up with pets and learned how much love pets give and how much care they need. For all four boys, music, travel and pets gave them special opportunities for creativity and communication.

Young people always yearn for independence. How to keep them from growing up too fast has forever been a challenge for parents. Living in community means rules for child, adolescent and adult alike. At some point or another, we must all learn respect, love, trust and rules. Freedom can exist only within rules and boundaries. A wholesome community provides a place for everyone.

Ideally, all children and adults would be healthy and perfect. When through chance or accident we're not, we remain just as precious and valuable to God and to the world. In community, we "all become vulnerable," writes Jean Vanier.

> There is a reciprocity, which communicates itself through the eyes and through touch. There is a sort of to-and-fro of love, a mutual understanding and respect which can lead people to share, laugh and celebrate together, or, in times of sorrow, to weep together. They speak heart to heart. Communion is founded on mutual trust in which a person gives to and receives from another that which is deepest and most silent in their being.[5]

## Spiritual journey

Franciscan spirituality consists of gospel living, community, and sharing with the poor – who, of course, include all challenged, marginalized and vulnerable persons. Franciscanism manifests itself in imitating Jesus with a joy that transcends worldly struggles, disappointments and fears. It has taught me to expect peace and joy in the daily events of my life. It has taught me to overcome the anxiety that accompanied me through much of my earlier years. Franciscan spirituality has given me the confidence to live fully.

But life is full of twists and turns – some of them so abrupt that one is caught off guard. The Church itself, God's vehicle on earth, is sometimes all too human, and wounds us, testing our patience to the limit. Then, too, our inner demons throw us off balance spiritually. Franciscanism has given me a means of coping with these difficulties. I amaze myself by finding a singing heart at the most unlikely times.

At my request, my sons have candidly revealed their current relationships with God to me. "The journey of faith demands that we let go of our image of God and our image of ourselves," says Franciscan author Father Richard Rohr. "But we can't do that in our head or on our own; it's done to us. The only thing we have to do is live, but live openly and honestly, letting the truth of the world get through to us."[6] I believe that my sons are living openly and honestly. They will absorb the truth as their journey progresses.

> Overall, I consider myself a spiritual person in that I see God in all aspects of life [says James]. Despite being a member of the CNN generation (which often depicts a pretty dark view of the world) and having seen poverty, violence and hatred first-hand while travelling with and without the military, I continue to see good almost everywhere. I think growing up within a family that dealt with disabilities daily gave me a unique perspective. It helped me see the positive during difficult times. Ironically, despite spending most of my adult life training for conflict as a Naval Officer, I feel very positive about my family's future.

> During my youth, I must admit that I lost faith from time to time, and Kevin being autistic was sometimes the source of my displeasure. I now think that most teenagers have internal demons that they must learn to deal with, and I think losing faith is very common at that age. As I grew older, I solved (through experience and time) most of my teenage issues, and also realized that Kevin was simply a biological statistic in a far greater whole. A statistic that my family, particularly my parents and younger brother, would have to deal with.

> When I was young [says Chris], I used to believe what I was taught in school: that God was a loving, caring and all powerful being who controlled all aspects of life and the world around us. And I also believed that God answered the prayers of the faithful. I can't think of anyone who would fit the title "faithful" more than my mother. I know that Mother prayed, joined prayer groups, and seemed to go (and take us along) to every shrine and prayer service she could think

of. I'm the only person I know whose mother went to the seminary.

I've never directly asked her, but I'm sure that the focus of her prayers and all the religious activity was in the hope of a cure for my brother.

Years have passed and my beliefs have changed. I now don't believe that God directly intervenes in the lives of the faithful. After all, I can't think of anyone who deserves that intervention more than my mother and my brother.

I grew up in a Catholic home, school and church, so God was a "given" to me [states Joel]. I know what I was taught, and praying was a routine. As an adult, I am fascinated by the idea of God, the stories of God, the ways other people respond to God, but I have not felt a true personal connection with God – at least in a spiritual way. I am in a questioning stage right now – seeking the answers that may never come.

And this is what Kevin says:

I believe that God is always with me and will always care for me. Sometimes I am angry with God for allowing me to be autistic. I wonder why he leaves me this way and doesn't cure me. I continue to hope that I will get better through medical ways. God works through natural means.

Faith is important to me because life has too many difficulties and is too short. I look forward to eternity with God and my parents and grandparents and brothers and their families and all our friends. In the meantime, God gives me the strength to carry on, and a measure of peace and happiness. I hope my family believes in God and finds peace in their lives.

It may surprise my sons that my spiritual journey needs ongoing adjusting as I struggle with my own demons. As they have observed, I am devoted to my faith and to the Catholic Church. I love the Church's devotions, sacraments, art, writings, tradition and scripture. I belong to its faith communities – my parish, my Franciscan fraternity, and the people of God. But I cannot help being affronted by the men-for-men leadership within my Church. After all, should not the Church be the model of justice towards men and women throughout the world? Shouldn't it set an example of disapproval for male-dominated nations where women and children are enslaved and abused?

Jesuit priest Richard Leonard notes that

> no papal teaching or Vatican document concedes at any stage that the church has been instrumental in maintaining a history of discrimination against women. In fact, the documents seem proud of the tradition of the church in relation to women, from the New Testament to the present day. However, what is striking about the New Testament women they name (for example, "Phoebe, a deacon of the church," Romans 16:11) is that in some cases their office in the church no longer exists; and some of the most important women are not mentioned at all. Also, when *Mulieris dignitatem*, for example, mentions the women of the tradition who "have shared in the church's mission" one of the common links between several of them is the confrontation they waged against male ecclesiastical authority or abuse in their day. This is certainly true for Birgitta of Sweden, Joan of Arc, Elizabeth Ann Seton, Mary Ward, Catherine of Siena and Teresa of Jesus.[7]

Leonard states further that

> John Paul II returns to the papal teaching of the 1950s by making Mary rather than Christ the direct model for all women. This revision is not helpful. By not following on in the teaching line of John XXIII and Paul VI, John Paul displaces the relationship women have directly with Jesus. Through baptism, Galatians says, we are all one *in Christ*. It is in and through Christ that all Christians find their human identity – male or female. It is in Christ and in relation to Christ that Mary found her dignity and vocation. This was the point of departure of the 1960s and 1970s that was so helpful. To return to Mary now, as the model for women, raises unnecessary questions christologically. For just as in Christ we all have our being, so in Mary we all – men and

women – find a model of being in Christ. Christ is for all and Mary is for all. One is the mirror and the other is an exemplary reflection.

Associated with this revision is Mary's promotion as virgin and mother, which is not helpful in an age that has seen women emerge strongly in social, political and professional leadership. Leaving aside the question of women's ordination to the priesthood, the modelling of women's options in terms of virginity and motherhood undermines a more hopeful reading of the Holy Spirit's action in the signs of the times. Again, John XXIII and Paul VI drew attention to this and encouraged women to reach their full potential in society.[8]

My own mother was a very spiritual person, totally loyal to the Catholic Church, but she lamented male ecclesial platitudes regarding women. "It's a man's world," she used to tell me when I was young, including the Church in that brush stroke, even as she clutched her rosary beads. As an older woman, Mother was angered by the injustice that drove one of my younger sisters to take her family of three sons and two daughters to Sunday Mass in another town when her local pastor forbade girls to serve on the altar. Apart from defending her daughters, my sister would not permit her sons to witness such disrespect for women.

Mother would agree with Rohr and be reassured by his words referring to men and women's participation in the Church: "The Incarnation had nothing to do with theology. It was rather about vulnerability, about letting go, about emptiness, about self-surrender – and none of that is in the head."[9] Jesus came for the salvation of all, and in his love, he valued men and women equally.

When I graduated from St. Peter's Seminary with a Master of Divinity degree, my husband, sons and their families attended the beautiful commissioning Mass and dinner. My eldest granddaughter, then not quite eight, told her mother that she wanted to be "a priest like Nana" when she grew up. I have never aspired to the priesthood, but I did feel called to be a deacon. For one tortured period during my studies at the seminary, I seriously discussed with my spiritual director a tantalizing pull towards the church of my Anglican grandmother.

Marie-Louise Ternier-Gommers, a Catholic laywoman living in Saskatchewan, speaks of *her* seminary experience, which somewhat parallels my own.

> Rather innocently and trustingly, and with deep love and desire, I opened myself wide to the learning and studying of the holy things of God and the Church: theology, liturgy, history, spirituality, sacraments, pastoral care. The learning helped me grow in my womanhood, and set ablaze a love and passion so great that the desire to serve in a leadership ministry grew and grew. In some ways I felt seduced, as if God had beckoned me under false pretense, for I soon joined the company of countless other women in history who experienced that same beckoning and could not respond fully within the existing church structures.... The emerging pain had to do with the faith community dimension of ministry, and with the reality of the communion of saints, with whom, as our church teaches, we remain connected across time. For among those saints were the legions of nameless women who spent their entire lives in painful invisibility yet in deep faithfulness to what they came to know as true and good.[10]

What saves me from disillusionment with the Church as a whole is my Franciscan family, my parish family, and my biological family. I am strengthened by the prayers, spirituality and community of my Secular Franciscan fraternity. I am encouraged by the men and women within the Church who defend the rights of all. I am gratified by the writings of Franciscan authors, male and female alike, who express sadness over the continued male dominance of the Church, but nonetheless retain faith and hope in the Church of Jesus Christ. I remind myself that even our Franciscan co-founder, Clare, resisted a Rule of Life imposed upon her by the pope of her day. Her persistence paid off with a papal change of heart, and as she lay dying, she received approval of her own Rule.

For the most part, my seminary experience was one of personal growth and joy. I went there to grow closer to God by learning more about God, God's love for all, and God's call to me. I met wonderful people with similar longings, and together we grew. The seminary instilled in me the need to share my gifts through my writing, and in service to my parish, my Franciscan Fraternity and St. Francis Advocates.

Last year, when American Franciscan priests were no longer able to serve the Sarnia area, our fraternity appointed me as Spiritual Assistant with the Region's approval. Despite recognizing the appointment as a privilege and honour, I accepted reluctantly. It was a time when I was heavily involved in parish work. So perhaps I resisted for selfish reasons, valuing personal space and time over an additional commitment. More likely, I feared having to deal with the fraternity's various spiritual leanings, preferring to stay neutral – and safe. But if this were the case, my imagination exceeded reality. The Fraternity welcomed my appointment with open enthusiasm and total support. After all, as Ron Rolheiser points out, a healthy theological community should find enough room in it for both Mel Gibson and Michael Moore.

> We cannot build either a society or a church with just liberals or just conservatives. To build community we need to work with more than just those who are like-minded. Any community or church built with just the like-minded is not worth belonging to because it reflects neither what's best inside the human spirit nor, for those of us who are Christians, the inclusive embrace of Christ.[11]

I have come to see that my role is simply to live in community, assisting my Franciscan brothers and sisters in their spiritual growth, just as they assist me. It is vanity on my part to believe that they expect more of me than I of them. We are on pilgrimage together, standing, as Rohr says, on "the shoulders of our forebears," and bearing "the burden of their sins and the fame of their holiness. They are an image of what we are, and we are an image of what they were. As you head out on the inner journey of faith, you will discover that you are exactly the same as them."[12]

On this journey, we are each mentor and seeker, sinner and saint, teacher and student. We are with God and in God.

# 4

# Addiction

**From Kevin's journal: Days 9 and 10 – Arrival in Nova Scotia**

*Day 9 – July 25, 1992 – Monastery, Havre Boucher, Mulgrave, and Port Hood*

"Can I see what you wrote?" asks Kevin at the motel that evening.

"Sure. Let me read it to you." I read Kevin the conversations I have transposed to date on my laptop.

"Did you have to say about the addictions?"

"We'll edit all this material before we publish your book," I promise, "and everything will have to be approved by you. However, I think that your story is more interesting and important because you have to deal with both autism and addictions. You will be an inspiration if you learn to overcome both."

"As far as I can tell, I guess that will do for now. Addictions are terrible. They make a person lose control of their right mind. They act like someone who's possessed of a demon."

"Addictions cause a lot of misery," I agree. "They are the reason you were sent to the Bob Rumball Centre."

"What are you so angry about?" I now ask. "I don't know what's wrong."

In time, Kevin calms down sufficiently to type, "I'm angry that you want to talk about Bob Rumball. I don't want to talk about it because it upsets me to remember those years. I was very unhappy then and it's difficult to think about. Why did you leave me there so long?"

"It's not like we left you there without bringing you home," I remind my son. "We visited you every third weekend, and usually took you home. And you were with us whenever we had holidays."

"I'm glad you took me home for holidays and weekends because that's all I lived for."

"I drove back and forth to Toronto through storms and all kinds of terrible weather and treacherous roads. I was desperate to see you. I missed you all the time."

"I'm glad to hear you say that."

"We didn't realize how aware you were, either, or that you were so lonely. We couldn't communicate with you." This had been in the frustrating days preceding facilitated communication.

"I knew you didn't know and that was very frightening. I thought I would be there forever."

"I would never have left you there forever. I was always telling you that."

"Yes, but I didn't believe you."

"I visited numerous institutions and residences and was constantly fighting with government ministries to get a residence started."

"I'm glad."

"I sent surveys all over Ontario. Hundreds of parents with autistic children wrote me letters telling of their despair and misery. Many of the children were already grown and had spent most of their lives in institutions."

"When are we getting to Cape Breton Island? Are we seeing mines? I hope we do. I want to see where the mine collapsed. I also wonder if they're still buried there."

"Some are still buried there. They tried to rescue them but they couldn't get them all out," I explain.

"That's terrible. Their families must feel sad. As far as I can tell, God is looking after them."

"I'm happy to be on this trip to the east," says Kevin later. "You're happy, too, and you and Dad are having a relaxing time. Are we going to visit the family graves today?"

"Are we going to have a good time at the graves?" he continues. "Are you happy I'm with you?"

Later still, at the Port Hood cemetery, where my maternal grandparents and several other of Kevin's relatives are buried, Kevin types, "When did they die?"

We point out the dates on the tombstones.

"As far as I can tell, that was a long time ago," says Kevin. "I feel proud to know that my great-great-grandparents were important people and part of this heritage."

In the evening Kevin types, "I'm wondering when we will have supper. I want coffee and dessert. I deserve it because I have had no butts all day."

*Day 10 – July 26, 1992 – Cabot Trail*

"Are you able to tell me what you were so agitated about last night?" I ask.

"I was, as far as I can tell, angry about many things such as being autistic and having addictions and being at the Bob Rumball Centre."

"It's understandable that you feel angry about those things from time to time."

"How do *you* feel about all those things?" asks Kevin.

"I get angry, too. I feel angry that I couldn't find a closer place for you all the time that you were at the Bob Rumball Centre. And I feel sad when I remember all the early years that I couldn't hold you and kiss you and comfort you because you wouldn't let me touch you without screaming and struggling and biting. I also feel guilty that I often gave absent-minded attention to your brothers because I was always worrying and fretting about you. Do you feel better when you can discuss your anger?"

"Yes, it helps when I can talk about it with you."

"Were the Bob Rumball staff kind to you?"

"As far as I can tell, most of them were, but a few of them did not seem to like me."

"Perhaps those would be the ones for whom it was just a job."

"Yes. They did it as a job for money."

"Who were your favourite counsellors?"

"Bonnie and Shari."

"Were you there long after Bonnie left?" Sometimes details, like when my sister, Bonnie, left for other employment, became a blur for me in those hectic years. Also I like to check Kevin's memory of past events in his life.

"Yes, I was there a long time."

"How long?" I know the answer to this, of course, but I was curious to know if Kevin did.

"As far as I can tell, several years."

"Do you feel that you were helped at all at the Bob Rumball Centre?"

"As far as I can tell, yes. Addictions got better."

"Do you remember your teacher at Bob Rumball?"

"She was very nice and I liked her."

"Do you feel better now?"

"Yes, I feel less angry."

"When you become agitated, do you want me to talk to you, or should I leave you alone?"

"As far as I can tell, you should leave me alone. I need time to think."

"Does prayer help?"

"Yes, as far as I can tell, prayer does help. I talk to Jesus and he comforts me."

"When I used to drive to Toronto by myself, I would call to you as I drove. I would say, 'Kevin! Kevin! I'm coming! I'm coming!' Could you feel me calling you?"

"No, I didn't know you were calling me, but I'm glad that you did. As far as I can tell, sometimes I could feel that you were coming and I would be happy."

"I was always thinking about you and missing you terribly," I say.

"I also had your love," says Kevin. "When I travelled with you, it made up for some of the lost time."

"I'm calm and relaxed today," he types later. "You did a good job of putting my childhood in perspective. Where are we going today?"

"Around the Cabot Trail."

"I'm happy we're seeing all the interesting places in Nova Scotia. And I'm glad we may be going to Newfoundland in two years. Where are we going next year?"

"We haven't decided yet."

"I want to know if you're taking me with you next year," he types.

"Of course we are."

"That's great."

"Why do you run ahead of us when we stop to see things?" I ask Kevin this at a bog boardwalk stop.

"I like to be independent. After all, I am 23 years old."

"What kind of souvenir do you want?"

"A ship."

"A carved wooden one?"

"Wood and sails like James has. It shouldn't cost too much."

Returning to our motel in the evening, I ask in dismay, "Why did you eat a butt?"

"It looked very tempting but it tasted terrible and I'm sorry I ate it. It wasn't worth it." It wasn't worth it because Kevin knows that he will be penalized by having no coffee for the rest of the day.

## Devastating obsessions

The summer of Kevin's twelfth birthday is a summer that might best be forgotten. That summer the lake had risen, eroding property and washing away sea walls. Up and down the shore, efforts were underway to stem the relentless damage caused by nature's excess. One of our neighbours was working on his embankment with a gas welder.

Since we could easily see Kevin from our yard, we would not always hurry to bring him home from any source of respite. Too late we became aware that Kevin was less interested in the machinery than in the gas fumes. He would have a tantrum when we pulled him away. Forbidden to leave our property, he turned his attention to our cars and lawnmower.

From there, his interest expanded to aerosol sprays, paints, varsol and insecticides. Inside the house, he rummaged endlessly through drawers and cupboards for things to sniff – cleaning solutions, correction fluid, perfumes, waxes. So obsessed did Kevin become with this activity that he would violently fight us off when we tried to remove a noxious substance from him.

Even at night we had no peace from Kevin's new obsession. As everyone slept, he would slip out into the night. Sixth sense (or was it Kevin's ever-vigilant guardian angel?) would waken me, and soon the whole family would be scouring the countryside with flashlights. We would find him semi-conscious beside some distant lawnmower or car.

One afternoon, a frightened, angry neighbour found Kevin not only in her garage, but in the trunk of her car. By this time, we were locking our own garage, and had purchased safety caps for our car's gasoline tank. But we could not lock up the entire county, and Kevin's search was relentless. At twelve, he had become hopelessly addicted to solvent sniffing.

Next we purchased contact alarms for the doors. Kevin outsmarted us by pushing out screens and breaking windows. The family was exhausted, irritable and miserable from lack of sleep. Kevin's brothers complained with growing outrage that they resented having such an impossible brother. The family's very survival seemed at stake.

We visited the Clark Institute in Toronto and were told that solvent sniffing was the most stubborn addiction because its reward was instant. In combination with autism, it would probably be untreatable. Inhalants are cheap and can be readily purchased off the shelf. They are a young or poor person's easiest route to intoxication.

The most commonly used inhalants are aromatic hydrocarbons. These include glue, gasoline, spray paint, paint thinners, lighter fluid, nail polish remover, and typewriter correction fluid. The effects are rapid, writes Dr. Allen Frances, and "consist of euphoria, a sense of invincibility, slurred speech, disinhibition, blurred vision, impaired judgement, visual distortion, dizziness, and loss of coordination. Higher doses can result in respiratory distress, stupor, coma, and death."[1]

If a person with autism has difficulty relating to others and an addicted person is indifferent towards others, what could be more isolating than a combination of the two? And what could be more difficult to escape from or treat?

Moreover, to have even a chance at effective treatment, the addicted person must first recognize the seriousness of the substance abuse problem, and then be motivated to change his deviant behaviour. Kevin seemed neither cognizant nor motivated.

And so we admitted defeat. After all our hard work and the wonderful progress Kevin was making, the family could no longer cope with him at home. More seriously, we feared that his life was in peril. As journalist Michael Swan wrote, "If you believe that everybody's life is equally precious, you will do two things. One, you will try to make sure they live through the night. And two...deal with the human being as [he] is now."[2]

Fortunately, we knew of a residence that might be appropriate as a temporary placement. My youngest sister, Bonnie, worked at the Bob Rumball Centre for the Deaf in North York, and had suggested that, since Kevin used sign language, it would be a good place for him. I had resisted heatedly, but now I phoned her for help.

Things happened quickly after that. Within a couple of weeks, Kevin was a resident of Bob Rumball some 300 kilometres from home. Family and friends were happy for us. They imagined that at last we could have a normal life. Jim and the boys wrapped their school days around themselves and carried on. For me, the days were endless gloom.

In the early days of Kevin's illness, I had written poems of hurt, anger, loneliness, abandonment and, sometimes, hope. Now I turned to poetry again, and penned my despair:

*October 19, 1981*

> I am not me
> when he is not here.
> My soul is dead.
> Fate has joined us
> with a permanent umbilical cord.
> Not a shackle,
> but a rainbow of dancing vibes.
> A rainbow of laughter and tears.
> As the rainbow vanishes
> without sun and rain,
> so does the song in my soul
> without him.

I consoled myself that in a year or two, a place closer to home would be found. But five years later, Kevin was still living in Toronto away from his family. By then we had established a routine of bringing Kevin home every third weekend. On Fridays I would drive to Toronto alone, and on Sunday afternoons, Jim, Kevin, Joel and I would drive back. Sometimes we spent the weekend in Toronto.

Whenever we would tell Kevin that he was going back to school, he became solemn and quiet. For the first year, we had to drag him moaning from the car whenever we reached the Bob Rumball Centre. Over time, he adapted to the routine and became more accepting.

It was altogether different when we picked Kevin up for a weekend or holiday home. Then, he jumped and clapped with delight. His eyes sparkled, he laughed aloud, and gave exuberant hugs and kisses. The residence staff would tell us that he had been in a state of barely controlled ecstasy all day.

On occasion, I had to call in a cancellation due to a winter storm. Once, while attempting to navigate snowy roads, I ended up in a ditch after narrowly missing a truck. "Oh, no!" a counsellor exclaimed over the phone. "However will we tell Kevin? He'll be *so* disappointed."

Through my own disappointment, I was reassured by the concern shown by the staff. I knew that Kevin was treated well at his residential school. Moreover, the programming was thorough and imaginative.

Nonetheless, as time passed, we continued to receive discouraging reports of Kevin's resistance to therapy. We were told that when the children's wing went on group outings, Kevin would race towards cars in the underground parking garage in order to quickly unscrew gas caps. Outside, he would break away from teachers and counsellors to snatch a discarded cigarette butt from the sidewalk. He would then chew and swallow the butt, resisting attempts to pry his mouth open. Staff also reported that he would sneak into the staff room to steal mugs of coffee at every opportunity.

Recently, I asked my other sons and my husband about their recollections of Kevin's years in Toronto. Their comments helped reassure me that the decision to send Kevin to the Centre was the right one – possibly the only one. They helped free me from a terrible guilt that has weighed upon me for a very long time.

> Although I do not remember much about the Bob Rumball facility, I do know that it was the best option available at the time [notes James, who was seventeen years old by then]. As far as I know, it provided the facilities and the dedicated attention that Kevin required. It was good to see Kevin when he returned home for visits, but it was always hard to see him return. I think my family (and I) felt guilty that we could not provide the best care for Kevin ourselves. I also

think, however, that outside intervention was required in order to attempt to effectively deal with an addicted autistic teenager.

I admit that, out of selfishness, I was relieved [comments Chris]. It meant that I wouldn't have to watch him anymore. I recall that prior to Kevin going to Bob Rumball, he was a handful and hard to keep an eye on. He was constantly running away to the neighbours' to sniff gas. My parents purchased locking gas caps for the neighbours' cars, and then he would sneak away to farther neighbours or into garages. When he went to Bob Rumball it was a break for me, and I was able to convince myself that Kevin was better off.

Later on, I began to have my doubts. His addictions seemed to be under better control. However, they always seemed to be just under the surface waiting to reveal themselves when an opportunity arose. I'm not sure that there were any other improvements occurring. It also became very apparent how extremely unhappy my mother was that Kevin was away, and I felt some guilt about this.

I don't recall anything in particular about Kevin's visits home. I always assumed that living at Bob Rumball was only a temporary arrangement, and that Kevin would be returning home someday.

Joel had just turned eight when Kevin went away.

Kevin was often my roommate at our house [says Joel], so there definitely was some loneliness for me when he went to Bob Rumball. Again, though, I was too young to know exactly what was happening to have any serious opinion on the matter at the time.

It became a routine, picking him up and dropping him off, so I guess I always had the optimistic outlook that we would see him soon. The longer visits such as Christmas would be tougher, but overall, looking back on it, I imagine it would have been much tougher for my mother and father. I still had the kid-naive outlook on the situation.

Jim adds,

I regretted he had to leave and the immense pain and work [driving] it caused Gloria. I still feel there was no choice. Kevin had a life-threatening addiction to gasoline. He would never have gone if Bonnie hadn't worked there. We had time for ourselves and the other boys (at least they couldn't use Kevin as an excuse), and Gloria found time, energy and the commitment to start St. Francis Advocates. So many good things came out of it despite the pain.

I always felt the Bob Rumball Centre was a decent, caring place, and at least we weren't taking him to an inappropriate institution, which would have been much worse.

## St. Francis Advocates: The early years

Although Kevin's addictions had not disappeared, our plans to bring him home continued. By the time Kevin turned fifteen, a group of concerned friends had joined us in establishing a non-profit organization called St. Francis Advocates. Our goal was to provide a local centre for autistic adults that would provide educational, vocational and residential services. The Ontario Society for Autistic Citizens was working with us, and government ministries were notified of our intentions.

## 1984 – The beginning

Everything begins with a dream. And dreams change with the tides of life. As our family lived on the shores of Lake Huron near the village of Camlachie, Jim and I discussed expanding our home into a residential school for adolescents with disabilities. I already had a busy Suzuki Music Studio there, and having parents and students coming and going seemed pleasantly normal. Music was always an important part of our family's existence. James started piano lessons with me at age four and Chris around the same age. For a couple of years they also studied violin with a teacher who came to our home. Then, when Joel was three years old, we decided to try out Suzuki violin lessons. My music teaching would never be the same.

The Suzuki method is based on Shinichi Suzuki's principle of *mother tongue*, in which he reasoned that young children learn speech by imitating their parents and the people around them. Only after they are capable of fluent speech are children taught to read, write and learn grammatical rules. Similarly, in the Suzuki method, children are first exposed to recorded music, which they are then encouraged to imitate on a musical instrument. The focus is on beautiful tone, proper posture and correct technique. Learning is acquired through listening, imitation and memory. A parent is required to attend lessons with the child and be the home teacher for the rest of the week. All aspects of the lesson are geared to the child, including the design of the instruments. Violins and cellos come in quarter, half and three-quarter sizes to accommodate the child's growth. Since pianos come in adult size only, young children are seated very high with feet supported.

So impressed was I by the method that I proceeded to teach Suzuki Piano to beginners in classes of three or four with parents or grandparents present. I attended Suzuki Piano Teacher Training Institutes in Kingston and London, Ontario. My teaching developed into a mixture of Suzuki and Conservatory, group and private lessons. The Sarnia-Camlachie Suzuki Piano Studio became so popular that I soon had to turn students away and transfer my senior students to traditional teachers. As well, I began to be approached by parents who had children with physical and developmental disabilities. These I always managed to accommodate because their accomplishments were of special delight to their families. Kevin loved music and took readily to the Suzuki method. At age ten, he played Bach's Minuet 2 in a small recital.

When Kevin left for treatment in Toronto for his addictions, the residential dream became more desperate. Regular letter writing to agencies and government ministries now became routine, with much impatient waiting in between replies. When responses did come, they often informed us that the matter was being sent on to another department.

I could relate to Luzina, Gabrielle Roy's heroine in *Where Nests the Water Hen*. Roy writes about Luzina receiving a long overdue letter explaining the reasons for delay in having the school she desired for her children.

> Surely the government had been put to a lot of trouble through her fault; Luzina blushed a little at what she had done. Moreover, the government explained, Luzina's letter addressed to the Gouvernement d'Instruction had taken a long while to reach the offices of the Department of Education and, among all its offices, that of Mr. Evans, who was in charge of precisely such requests as Luzina had made.[3]

But, like Luzina, I was motivated by a necessity-driven faith. Kevin *needed* to return to his community, and persistence *had* to bring results. However, I eventually came to realize that the residence on the lake was not to be. In fact, as the days and months and years slipped by, it became apparent that it would not be an adolescent residence at all, but an adult one.

Three years into my letter-writing campaign, I began to entertain the thought that perhaps I could not do this single-handedly. I turned to my Secular Franciscan community to pray for the project, which then became *their* project. Next I asked a Franciscan friend, Reta Mitro, to help me. Reta was intrigued by the project. She and I soon envisioned a rural residence, with gardens and animals, maybe a greenhouse, and operated in the manner of L'Arche homes.

L'Arche began in 1964 when Jean Vanier and Father Thomas Philippe invited two men with mental handicaps to live with them in Trosly, France. From this first community, born in the Roman Catholic tradition, many other communities throughout the world have developed in various cultural and religious traditions. Core members and their attendants live, work, pray and celebrate together. In Vanier's words, "Each person, according to his or her vocation, is encouraged to grow in love, self-giving and wholeness, as well as in independence, competence and the ability to make choices."[4]

In August 1984, we met with Brother Anthony VandenHeuvel of the Brothers of St. Louis and outlined our dream to him. We explained that we wished to dedicate the project to St. Francis of Assisi because Francis was noted for his gentleness, his appreciation of creation in its entirety, and his acceptance of the "lepers" of society.

Brother Anthony immediately became interested and presented the idea to Bishop John Sherlock of the London (Ontario) diocese. The bishop readily endorsed the project and promised to pray for our success, but he did not offer to help us establish our residential dream, as we had dared to hope. We continued our quest.

During the fall, Reta and I visited L'Arche communities in Stratford and Toronto and admired their spirituality and lifestyle. We wondered if they might expand into our area, and in turn were asked if we could do some of the groundwork, such as finding property and our own residential director. Since Jim and I were still somewhat interested in operating a residence, I felt a brief flicker of optimism. It was quickly extinguished when it was then explained that a residential director required two years of live-in experience at a L'Arche facility.

Next we enlisted the assistance of the Ontario Society for Autistic Children. Jim had been president of the London chapter since 1982, as well as a director on the provincial board. He and I were also active members of the Windsor chapter. Many of these parents were involved in residence searches of their own, and we were able to share ideas, encouragement and lobbying.

## 1985 – The founding board

By June 1985, others had graciously accepted the invitation to join us, and St. Francis Advocates became an established organization. The first Board of Directors consisted of nine dedicated friends.[5] Reta and I were president and vice-president respectively. Reta's sister-in-law, Mary Mitro, became a most diligent secretary-treasurer, taking over much of my letter writing. Fortunately, in those early days, she had no idea of the years of writing yet to come.

The nine of us attended workshops and conferences on autism, and visited group homes near and far. We collected information on hobby farms, weaving, greenhouses, and anything else that might enrich the lives of our future tenants.

We wrote to Canada Mortgage and Housing, requesting that St. Francis Advocates be immediately considered for housing assistance, and met with the Ministry of Community and Social Services. Our friends Gerald Bloomfield, provincial president of the Ontario Society for Autistic Children, and his wife, Elizabeth, both professors at the University of Guelph, spoke to our board and encouraged us to remain tenacious in pursuing our goal.

In December 1985, the provincial office received a sobering letter from the Ministry of Community and Social Services stating that there was no identified population diagnosed by the classification "autistic adult." Only the classification of "childhood autism" or "infantile autism" was recognized. Adults would not be treated as autistic adults, but rather as having "autistic thinking" found in schizophrenic thought patterns.

In the letter, the ministry noted that counselling services for schizophrenia were offered through the Ministry of Health, while life skills programs and vocational training were provided by associations for the developmentally handicapped. The "limited number of identified autistic adults" could be accommodated by existing service programs. In other words, forget trying to start something new.

## 1986 – Year of triumphs and trials

The St. Francis Board persevered, continuing to send letters to the ministries of Housing and of Community and Social Services requesting group home application. It was now 1986.

Then some good news! The United Way of Sarnia Lambton awarded us a grant of $7000 through its demonstration and development fund. From this we could buy office equipment and supplies, pay for advertising, publicity and consultation costs, and cover some travel expenses. Inspired, we drew up a constitution and pressed for charitable donation status and incorporation. Our official title became St. Francis Advocates for the Autistic and Developmentally Disabled Inc.

To further meet ministry requirements, we sent a needs survey to numerous institutions and associations. The response indicated that there were more than a hundred autistic persons in area institutions. We also sent out a questionnaire to families through the *Ontario Autism* newsletter. Replies included the previously mentioned personal and heart-wrenching letters from parents, praying that we might help them.

Over the late summer and fall, the Ministry of Housing began sending us start-up funding but reminded us that a commitment from the Ministry of Community and Social Services was necessary before capital funding would be released. For its part, the Ministry of Community and Social Services continued to request updated copies of our constitution, board of directors, management rationale, draft organizational plan, needs assessment results, and possible housing sites. We kept the paper flowing.

The Housing ministry continued to move forward. On September 5, we learned that our proposal for eight social-housing units had been selected for preliminary consideration under the 1987 non-profit housing program allocations!

In late October, the board met with Michael Byrne, programme supervisor from the Ministry of Community and Social Services' Windsor area office to discuss approval of a site in Sombra, Ontario, as well as staffing, programming and funding. We were cautiously optimistic.

But in November we met with the London area office and were presented with a totally different concept: instead of a rural community of individuals, we should be looking at one person, Kevin, and building around his needs. The St. Francis Advocates Board felt that this would be unrealistic for our current goals and the progress we had made with the Ministry of Housing.

On a personal note, I was terrified that this could be a major setback to Kevin returning home from Toronto. I asked the Secular Franciscans locally and provincially to pray with renewed fervour for the project's success.

Unaware of our latest setback with the Social Services ministry, the Housing ministry sent us another funding payment, reminding us that a commitment from Ministry of Community and Social Services was necessary before capital funding would be released.

In December, the Ministry of Community and Social Services agreed that "the autistic are a group who have been overlooked." Funds would be made available for them. They did not say when these funds would materialize.

### 1987 – Year of politics

By 1987, Kevin had been in treatment in Toronto for five-and-a-half long years. In early February, the Ministry of Housing informed us that, due to the lack of response from the Ministry of Community and Social Services, St. Francis Advocates would not be receiving funds for housing units under the 1987 program. We were devastated.

A few days later, the board met with the Social Services ministry to discuss this unhappy turn of events. Jim and I insisted that Kevin return to our community at once and that suitable arrangements be made to facilitate this process.

The St. Francis Board reassured me that they would continue fighting for a residence, but I feared they were becoming as worn out as I was.[6] It was time for political activism. We appealed for help to the Ontario Society for Autistic Citizens and to our Lambton and Sarnia members of Parliament. We continued to send forms, letters and applications to both ministries.

The Ontario Society for Autistic Children had changed its name to the Ontario Society for Autistic *Citizens* to more accurately reflect its mandate. In a change of policy, the society had recently decided to permit the establishment of new chapters. We were encouraged to start a chapter in Sarnia. By the summer of 1987, the newly chartered Sarnia-Lambton Chapter was already involved with fundraising, public relations activities, and political lobbying. Not surprisingly, Jim was president, I was secretary, and St. Francis Advocates took out a membership.

In August, the Ministry of Housing announced once again that the Advocates had received approval to develop residential housing. As before, their funding was provisional on operational funding from the Ministry of Community and Social Services.

Also in August 1987, Kevin returned home! The Social Services ministry gave us a generous allowance of 20 home-support hours per week, and St. Patrick's High School in Sarnia was awaiting his arrival in September.

**Spiritual journey**

Often our spiritual journey plunges us into darkness. The darkness can take many forms. Addiction is one such darkness, and has been with us as long as we humans have had time to seek pleasure. "Who has woe? Who has sorrow? Who has strife? Who has complaining? Who has wounds without cause? Who has redness of eyes?" asks the book of Proverbs rhetorically. The answer: "Those who linger late over wine.... At the last it bites like a serpent, and stings like an adder. Your eyes will see strange things, and your mind utter perverse things. You will be like one who lies down in the midst of the seas" (Proverbs 23:29-34).

Jean Vanier also addresses the darker side of pleasure.

> Pleasure is a very ambiguous reality. There are dangerous pleasures, deadly pleasures, and those which create a need, a habit (drugs, for example, not only imprison the person in habit but also within a world of imaginary excitement, and, at the same time, begin to destroy the brain). Such pleasures impede true spiritual growth. They keep one from knowing reality, from knowing one's true needs and the needs of others, from loving other people and from making an effort in the struggle for peace and justice. The pursuit of pleasure for oneself implies a certain indifference towards others; and, when the seeking becomes total, it cuts a person off from others completely.[7]

Absorbed in their relentless pursuit of narcissistic pleasure, addicts remain hooked despite painful consequences. Thus, rather than give up his addictions, Kevin remained far from home, separated from the family he loved.

Kevin was, and still could readily become, addicted to caffeine, nicotine and inhalants. All are seriously addictive. Caffeine is "by far the most frequently used psychoactive substance in the entire world," says Frances.[8] Since it is so universally enjoyed and accepted, we allow Kevin to enjoy one or two cups a day, as do we. Sometimes, however, immediately after having coffee, he begins to hysterically demand more. A firm reminder that such behaviour is unacceptable, or the suggestion that perhaps he should not have coffee at all, usually brings him to his senses.

Nicotine is another matter – and especially distressing since Kevin likes his in the form of used cigarette butts. It is the most addictive of all substances, with its unpleasant withdrawal symptoms probably explaining the high rates of relapse among those who attempt to forgo it. "These begin within a few hours of nicotine deprivation and include intense cravings, anxiety, difficulty concentrating, agitation, depressed mood, increased appetite, decreased heart rate, and insomnia," Frances explains.[9]

As for inhalants, their availability and the rapid onset of their effects are the lure. All addictive drugs produce alterations in the brain that increase susceptibility to relapse and cravings even years after successful detoxification. Over time, an addicted individual requires the addicting substance just to feel normal. The pleasure pathway in the brain, the "dopamine reward circuit," is connected to areas that control memory, emotion and motivation.

But eventually the dopamine circuit becomes blunted. The drug "simply pushes the circuit back to normal, boosting the user out of depression but no longer propelling him or her towards euphoria. By repeatedly supplying the body with the substance, a new state of 'normal' is created, causing the person to continue using the substance in order to feel normal," reports Jane Brody.[10]

On a positive note, these changes in the brain, although long lasting, are not permanent. With the proper therapy and support systems, recovery is attainable. Kevin, in fact, has made great strides in conquering his additions. "Kevin's addiction to sniffing gasoline was major and life threatening," notes my husband, Jim. "It's the most serious addiction known and the hardest to treat. I am so thankful that he seems to be over it since he returned from Toronto."

But Kevin is prone to relapses when it comes to ingesting cigarette butts. Moreover, when he has such a relapse his overall behaviour deteriorates. This is not surprising, since, in deacon Roy Barkley's words, "an addict's quest to avoid reality results in arrested emotional development. Preserving the emotional traits of a thwarted adolescent, he becomes unable to communicate honestly, and creates a life of denial and evasion."[11]

Why did Kevin fall into the trap of addiction to begin with? Persons with disabilities are susceptible to acquiring various addictions to fill their uneventful lives and distract them from their many frustrations. It is therefore necessary to find the empty place within such individuals, and help them fill the emptiness in a meaningful way.

As our son James explains,

> I think addiction was an escape for Kevin. You try being autistic for a while. Many non-disabled people fall prey to addictions, and often outside intervention, continuous counselling, and a large support network are the only things that get them through.
>
> As far as Kevin is concerned, I can't imagine being considered an outcast from society, not understanding (for the most part) my environment every minute of every day, being at the mercy of those around me, and probably feeling very much alone very much of the time. Given those circumstances, I think that I'd be sniffing gas, glue, and whatever else I could get my hands on.

Chris says,

> I can appreciate how someone can find a substance that makes them feel good temporarily (such as sniffing gas), appealing. And I can appreciate how someone would want to experience that good feeling over and over until they become addicted.
>
> I'm not an expert on addictions, but I can see how this could be disastrous for someone like Kevin. It's my understanding that for someone to kick a habit like this, they would have to develop the fortitude and willpower to stop sniffing, and to make it through the withdrawal period and ongoing crav-

ings, while telling themselves that enduring the pain now will pay off with a better addiction-free life in the future. If Kevin does not see the negative long-term consequences of addiction, it must be almost impossible not to give into his temptations.

Kevin's difficulties are compounded by the obsessive-compulsive component inherent in autism. It is recognized that repetitive behaviours accompany obsessive thoughts, and both are driven by underlying anxiety. Dealing with the cause of the anxiety is therefore essential. Kevin worries and frets about his future. He worries about what will become of him when Jim and I die. He envisions a life of dependence, tedium, and possibly neglect stretching before him.

We remind him that we constantly have his future in mind. To begin with, that is what St. Francis Advocates is all about. Then there are his brothers who will always have his best interests at heart. We hope he will gain more independence before we die. Kevin is relieved and happy to be told these things, but his security is fragile and needs to be reinforced regularly.

Without planned efforts to enrich life in areas where it has been stunted by addiction, "relapse is almost certain and the spiritual growth of true recovery is almost impossible," Barkley says.[12]

Joel addresses the issue of relapse.

With addictions, temptation is key, and I feel there is too much temptation (cigarette butts) for Kevin, causing his willpower to crack.

I also feel that maybe everyone takes it for granted that Kevin is cured. If you have an alcoholic relative, you are always cautious about alcohol around him. Similarly, a 100–per cent smoke-free environment would benefit Kevin greatly.

Unfortunately, cigarette butts are strewn about in many public places. Kevin himself must recognize that he has a problem and be motivated to resist relapse. "After an addict is well established in recovery, his initiative, sense of competence, and feeling of security in God's hands insulate him against relapse," says Barkley.

There is, however, a stage between early sobriety and the self-assurance of mature recovery that is especially dangerous. Initially, the addict discovers new depth and pleasure in many aspects of his life, "but the high wears off, and the addict enters a period of new recognition that life is not perfect, after all," Barkley adds.[13]

A pastoral approach to the addict's condition "should be strongly affirmative and should stress the hope for improvement, not the damage that has been done." The addict is only too cognizant of his weaknesses." He needs help to put them in perspective. Then he can keep them in the back of his mind as a motive for good without wearing them as an anchor.[14]

Once again it comes down to nurturing a sense of dignity and purposefulness, and allowing for the healing grace of God's love.

# 5

# Resources

**From Kevin's journal: Day 11**

Day 11 – July 27, 1992 – Fort Louisbourg and Sydney

"Did you write about our trip?" asks Kevin.

"Yes, I copied down everything from your organizer," I say. "Your first book should be finished this summer."

"But when will we find time to do it?"

"We've been doing it all along. What's the story on butts today?"

"I will not eat any."

"That's super," I respond with cautious hope.

"Yes. I have my rather bad-tasting tobacco."

"Is it worse than the taste of butts?" I ask. After all, we're comparing aromatic pipe tobacco to used cigarette butts.

"Yes."

"Still, it's not as unhealthy as a butt."

"It's awful knowing that butts are poisonous and, as far as I can tell, contaminated."

"That's right. You can never tell what germs you might be picking up."

"Where are we going today?"

"To Fort Louisbourg."

"As far as I can tell, that should be fun."

"It *will* be fun."

As we stand outside Fort Louisbourg, Kevin types, "What are we doing here?"

"This is about history."

"I'm not really interested in history."

"But it's one of the subjects you will be studying in school in the fall. This should help you with it."

"As far as I can tell, I will try to understand," he says. But later, Kevin types, "I'm angry that we're here."

"But it's so interesting," I protest.

"As far as I can tell, it will be boring."

"Wait till you see the people in costumes of the eighteenth century, and everything replicated as it was then! I'm sure you'll like it."

"I hope so."

"What year are we in now?" I ask.

"1992."

"And what year is being replicated here?"

"1744."

"That's right! And what happened here?"

"As far as I can tell, the French were defeated by the British. So why did they build it?"

"So we could experience what it was like to be here in 1744."

"As far as I can tell, I've seen it before," says Kevin.

"But you were very young then." It was at least ten years since we had last been there with our sons.

"I still remember it."

"You can't remember it very well, and besides, it has changed a lot since then."

"I have seen other forts."

"Will you try to behave appropriately?"

"I will try to be interested. When will we leave?"

"After we've seen everything."

"As far as I can tell, perhaps it will be fine. As far as I can tell, it will perhaps be fun."

"Certainly."

"This is very strange," comments Kevin, after we are challenged by a guard in period costume at the fort entrance.

"Why did Dad lie about us being French?"

"Dad was playing the game so they would not think we were English spies. What did the guards say?"

"They gave us rules to follow," says Kevin.

Shortly afterwards, I ask him, "Why are those men playing musical instruments and singing, while a prisoner is being dragged off?"

"It was entertaining to see someone punished."

"Yes, and they used to get *really* excited when there was a hanging."

"That is not very compassionate."

"For sure. Are you enjoying yourself?"

"Yes. It's very realistic. Are we going to eat here?"

"Yes." We are now on the sidewalk outside an eatery.

"Then will we leave?"

"After a while."

"We have seen most of the things. Where are we staying tonight?"

"Sidney again."

"That's good. I'm tired. Why are we waiting?"

"We have to wait for a place in the restaurant."

"I hope those people don't get in ahead of us."

"They won't. Everybody has to wait his turn."

Once inside the fort's restaurant, I ask, "What would you like from the menu?"

Kevin examines the menu carefully. Finally, he requests, "Soup, meat pie, and coffee."

"What do you think about this place?"

"It is unusual how they ate. It's very authentic and interesting. As far as I can tell, they had difficult and dangerous lives."

When we are ready to leave the Fort, we walk towards the bus area. Suddenly, Kevin dashes ahead, and boards a departing bus. Tired as we are, Jim and I run after the bus, waving our arms and shouting. To our relief the bus driver stops and waits for us to catch up.

I find a seat beside Kevin and ask, "Kevin, why did you run ahead and board the bus without us?"

"I wanted to go alone," he replies.

"Your dad and I had to chase the bus, and it almost didn't stop for us!"

"Yes. That was my intention."

"What would you have done then?" I ask.

"I would have waited at the other end."

"Would you not have been frightened?"

"No, I would not have."

"Where would you have gone?"

"I would have waited in the building."

"We wouldn't have known where to look."

"I would have found you. I wanted to do it all by myself."

Later in the day, Jim asks Kevin, "Do you hear the foghorn?"

"Yes."

Jim: "What is it for?"

Kevin: "When ships can't see through the fog, the horn tells them where the rocks are."

Jim: "You know so much, Kevin, I think you really could handle the bus by yourself."

Kevin: "Why did you put in about the bus?"

Jim: "It's still fresh in my mind."

Kevin: "I want to be more independent."

Jim: "Do you want to travel with us?"

Kevin: "Yes, but I want to do some things without you."

Jim: "What kind of things?"

Kevin: "I would like to live in an apartment some day."

(Living to see ever-increasing independence in our son is something that we dearly desire.)

We've availed ourselves of numerous superb resources in Kevin's life to date, and we won't hesitate to turn to them in the future. My biggest fear, in fact, is that I'll miss something.

## The Integra Foundation and other resources

The years between Kevin's sixth and twelfth birthdays were years of hard work and optimism. During that period, we worked with the Integra Foundation which, at that time, was funded by the Ministry of Health. Now called the Geneva Centre for Autism,[1] it is funded by the Ministry of Community and Social Services. This unique program for autistic children consisted of an intensive summer camp experience followed by home visits from Integra staff throughout the year.

In the spring of 1975, when Kevin entered their program, Integra was planning its second summer at Camp Towhee in Haliburton. In order to have one's child accepted, a family agreed to participate in a demanding home-and-school program involving behaviour analysis methods.

The program consisted of a month at camp and an intensive home-school follow-up program throughout the school year. Under the guidance of the Geneva Centre, the whole family learned sign language and Kevin was taught to read, play the piano and do many other activities. Our home was plastered with charts and graphs, but optimism had replaced despair.

Although Joel was only two years old when we started working with Integra, our involvement continued through his early years. He says, "I only have limited snapshot reflections of Integra, and of the summer camps."

Chris remembers, "At the time I was young and I was under the impression that these people were checking up on our family, and I didn't like it one bit. To this day, I'm not really sure who they were and what their purpose was."

Although they worked us relentlessly, and our walls were papered with time-consuming projects and charts, we adults loved those enthusiastic, dedicated people. The children may have been somewhat less enthused at living in a laboratory environment.

So remarkable was the change in Kevin after his first Integra summer camp, we were ecstatic when he was chosen again the following summer from among the applicants. It was like winning the lottery, and I recorded the experience for posterity:

> August 1976. Camp begins on August 12. All campers are to be settled in by 4:00 p.m., so we have been up since 6:00 a.m. My mother, in fact, has phoned long distance to ensure our prompt departure. After many false starts, we are on our way by 8:00 a.m., a tumultuous carload of two adults, four boys, a dog and a cat.
>
> There is an air of restrained excitement about our journey. Even Kevin is infected by it. Usually calm and content in moving cars, he is rocking back and forth, sitting intently on the edge of the back seat. We have explained to him that he is returning to Camp Towhee, but cannot be sure that he understands.
>
> Kevin is probably unaware of his good fortune in being accepted for two consecutive summers. Of the twenty children who attended last summer, only eight are included in

this year's twenty. The Integra Foundation, which operates the three-week camp and its follow-up program, is funded by the Children's Services Branch of the Ontario Ministry of Health. The project is still an experimental one, and its expansion will depend on tangible results. In a time of inflation and scrimping, who but the families of autistic children will view such a program as a priority?

Several hours later, we are driving down the long, primitive lane that winds through the woods to a cozy collection of cabins snuggling alongside a small lake. The scene, so serene and beautiful, immediately reassures us that the setting, at least, could not be improved upon.

We come to a stop and Kevin, ignoring our shouts to wait, leaps from the car, his face bright with joyful recognition. As he rushes towards the kitchen compound, we exchange glances of relief, and follow behind, toting his duffle bags. Inside the dining hall, we are introduced to his counsellor, Kris, and attempt to introduce her to Kevin. But he is puzzled, expecting last year's Deedee, and tries to walk around the young woman. Kris gently persists in leading him to his cabin, with all of us in tow.

Now there are chats with more of the staff: the director, nurse, swim instructor, cabin co-ordinator, float counsellor, and teachers of language, classroom, music and physical education. Many are new, but some are old friends. Later, a few glimpses of Kevin, who averts his gaze whenever we manage to catch it, and we are homeward bound. I am slightly disturbed that he was not around for goodbye kisses when we left.

"What do you think he'll be like when we pick him up this year?" asks Christopher. "Remember last year when James said, 'It's just like getting a new brother?'"

I remember, and hope wells within me. Last summer the camp achieved the impossible. In three short weeks, Kevin learned the beginnings of sign language, general obedience, and several basic self-help skills. He could dress himself, wash, brush his teeth, and his table manners put his brothers to shame. Incredulous, we took him home anticipating a productive year.

But his progress had not measured up to our expectations. He had behaved appropriately in the special education classroom, and his teachers were pleased with his compliance, but he had demonstrated minimal academic acquisitions. Moreover, his behaviour at home had gradually deteriorated under our waning vigilance. Our main success had been in learning a considerable number of sign gestures as a family.

And now, thank God, we are getting another chance. This time, we vow, we will not be lulled into complacency. We will commit ourselves totally to the hard work demanded of a behaviour modification program.

*Two weeks later*

It is August 25, visiting day for Cabin 4. Kevin's brothers and pets are at their grandparents', and Jim and I are having coffee in the camp dining hall with four sets of likewise-anxious parents. We exchange pleasantries, but tension electrifies the room. Finally, we are led to a rustic classroom, and invited to sit on benches around the walls.

Years of one-way expressions of love have taught us not to expect exuberant greetings from our autistic offspring. Not expecting, but ever ready to accept, the mothers and fathers watch hopefully. Occasionally, one sees a tentative wave or a silently mouthed "Hi" from the audience. It's as if each parent is embarrassed to expose his naïveté by openly courting recognition from an autistic son or daughter.

But the children steadfastly pursue their tasks. There is no showing off in this classroom. They sit in a giant circle on the floor, each child with his own counsellor. There are, as well, group leaders and head instructors. The atmosphere is pleasant. One feels that these students are responding to the faith placed in them by the camp. Rarely, if ever before, have they had the opportunity to experience pride in a job well done. If only camp could last forever.[2]

"I was very appreciative that people took an interest in providing care for Kevin," says James. "Those who dedicate their lives in attempting to help developmentally disabled people are exceptional people."

Jim agrees: "I thought all of that was excellent, and we should be glad we experienced it."

During the years of inspiration from Integra, Kevin continued to receive speech therapy at the Children's Treatment Centre. The Centre's speech therapists were well qualified and did excellent work. Several individuals on staff had always been genuinely friendly and supportive. Even in the painful early days, Kevin benefited from the attention and care they lavished upon him. The Centre's director was succeeded by one who accepted parents as partners, and our relationship with the Centre improved.

The wife of the new director, Diana Wilson-Wright, came to our home regularly as a volunteer to work with Kevin. She developed a close relationship with everyone in our family. Diana was sensitive, enthusiastic and creative, and she became a personal friend.

Pictures taken during this time show Kevin smiling proudly with his First Communion class, Kevin baking cookies with his after-school tutor and some neighbourhood children, Kevin posing only somewhat reluctantly with his three brothers in a formal portrait.

## Spiritual journey

During the Integra years, we had great hope that Kevin would achieve normal or near-normal independence. But as Kevin's journal entries indicate, at 23 he still could not be out of our sight without causing alarm.

Looking back on the memory of Kevin boarding the bus alone gives my heart a twist. I see myself finding a seat beside Kevin on the crowded bus and asking, "Kevin, why did you run ahead and board the bus without us?" I remember being surprised, and yet not surprised, by his response: "I wanted to go alone."

I remember that, although our hearts were pounding with the fright, we were proud of his intelligence and, at the same time, sad for his inabilities. Kevin was more impulsive in his twenties than he is now in his thirties. He is more responsible in many ways, and far less inclined to become agitated. His patience and humility are admirable, and a model for those of us who do not have his limitations.

When family or friends gather, he sits quietly on the sidelines, listening to the chatter and activity around him. Occasionally, he will frown and look unhappy. But, more often, he smiles and seems delighted to be silently present. He does not initiate conversation, but always has plenty to say when asked.

Kevin spends hours waiting for others to decide what will take place on a given day, where he will go and what he will do. Only when specifically asked what he wishes to do will he type a request. Since the fall of 1994, Kevin has had computers with a choice of six synthesized voices – first a LiteWriter and, more recently, a Dynavox. He is very particular about the voice that should speak for him. Finding helpful resources continues to be a ritual in our lives. Many resources, spiritual and otherwise, can be found in the secular field.

When asked, Kevin does not hesitate to name several resources that enrich his life:

Travelling is the most important thing to me because it stimulates all my senses and I can be with people I like. My family is a great resource. They are always looking after my best interests. St. Francis Advocates is a good resource for autistic people and their families. They keep up to date on everything that's new. My house is a nice place to be when I am not with my family. I like the staff and the Daves and all the interesting things we do.

Animals are nice to have around. They're funny and smart and they like when I come home. Nature is a wonderful creation of God. The earth is beautiful and awesome.

I have a special group of new friends that I can use facilitated communication with. They understand the way I feel and we can share our common problems and concerns.

The most special resource is my parents. Now that my grandparents are dead, my parents are very important to me and I am afraid of what will become of me when they die. Spirituality gives meaning to my life. Knowing God is with me all the time gives me the courage to make it through each day when there is nothing else going for me. Heaven is where everyone is equal.

I know that I am as important and valuable as everyone else but others don't see me that way. They think I am not aware that they don't value me and they don't know I have thoughts and feelings like them. Until recently most people thought this. Now more people know I'm smart because I am acting more normal. When this book comes out it will surprise lots of people who are unaware of the prisons we are in, and think we are as we seem physically.

Franciscan spirituality is an important resource for Kevin. As he points out philosophically, "Francis liked people who were outcasts like me. He lived with people who were different, and some of them were holy. He was happy with whatever God sent his way. Clare was perhaps calmer than Francis. She stayed in a convent with her sisters, and worked and prayed. We should talk about her presence in Assisi and my experience there." (In Chapter 14 we will look at Kevin's Assisi experience.)

Franciscan spirituality is a vital resource for all the world. It is a paradox, writes Sister Frances Teresa,

> that all those years learning to love the crucified Christ made Clare into what we long to be: a happy woman. While her letters are remarkable for their spiritual quality and depth, they also glowed with a simple happiness which catches at our hearts. When she first talked to Francis, an insight into joy opened to her.[4]

Franciscans are people of joy and hope, knowing God is with us. Gradually, we have come to know that, despite our brokenness and sin, we cannot stop God from loving us.

# 6

# Relationships

**From Kevin's Journal: Day 12**

"Where are we going today?" asks Kevin.

"Sightseeing in Nova Scotia," I reply.

"That's great."

"You had a good history lesson yesterday."

"Yes. I learned about the French and the British fighting over Fort Louisbourg in order to have control over Canada."

"Exactly. Will you be able to avoid butts today?"

"I will be okay because I am calm."

"And you weren't calm yesterday?"

"As far as I can tell, I was not calm."

Later, as we were watching the news on TV, I ask Kevin, "What seems to be the trouble in Iraq?"

"Saddam Hussein won't let the U.N. inspect the arsenal and there may be war."

"What kind of a person is Saddam Hussein?"

"Wicked. Are we going to be on Cape Breton much longer?" Kevin slips in what's really on his mind.

"Only a couple of hours."

"I wish we could stay here," says Kevin.

"So do I, but we've had a good time."

"Where are we staying tonight?"

"Somewhere around Sherbrooke. We don't have a reservation for any place in particular."

"Good."

Sometime later, when we're driving in the car, Kevin's rocking and agitated behaviour forces us to pull over to the side of the road. "What is wrong?" I ask. "Why were you clapping?"

"I'm angry that we're heading back towards the west."

"We still have almost two weeks left on our holiday, and we will stay in Nova Scotia even though we are leaving Cape Breton."

"That's good. I still wish we could travel forever."

"We all wish that, but we have to go back and work so that we can look forward to our next holiday."

"I guess I will have to accept that."

Jim: "Would you like me to buy a tape with Cape Breton fiddle music?"

"It's fine but I would rather have one with songs."

Jim: "We already have one like that."

"Get another one. I don't like just fiddle music."

When we stopped at Rita's Tea House and Gift Shop, Kevin inquires, "Who is Rita?"

"Rita McNeil. She's a well-known Cape Breton singer," I say.

"I hope so."

That evening, Kevin seems withdrawn. "Tell me how you're feeling, honey," I encourage. "What's wrong?"

"I feel sad and lonely. I wish I wasn't autistic. I want to be normal like other people."

"Do you often feel sad?"

"Yes. I feel depressed."

"What do you get depressed about?"

"Being autistic."

"Can you tell me how you feel?"

"I feel fearful and anxious."

"About what?'

"Being alone. Having no friends. Not being able to get married."

"What other things do you think about?"

"I would like to be able to get a university degree and be a writer."

"You should be able to do that."

"I hope so."

"Anything else?"

"I would like a house and a car, and live on a farm by a lake on Cape Breton."

"That would be nice, all right. Would anyone live with you?"

"My wife and children."

"Would there be animals on the farm?"

"Yes, a dog, calves, horses, sheep, goats and pigs."

"That would be a lot of work. Who would do it?" I ask.

"I would have hired men and make money writing so that I could pay them."

"It sounds like you've put a lot of thought into this."

"Yes. I do a lot of thinking," says Kevin.

"Today is such a rainy day, Kev, that I think it contributes to depression. I've read that heavy molecules in the air actually weigh us down."

"That's probably true. I feel much better when the sun shines."

"Depression is something everyone feels sometimes to one degree or another. But some people have more depression than others. I used to get depressed more often than I do now."

"Do you still sometimes get depressed?"

"Yes, I do."

"As far as you can tell, what makes *you* depressed?" Kevin asks me.

"Usually there doesn't seem to be any rhyme or reason to it," I say.

"It's the same with me. As far as I can tell, some days are just depressing."

"What per cent of the time do you feel depressed?"

"40 per cent."

"So you're happy most of the time."

"Happy or at least content."

"But sometimes you're not."

"Yes, sometimes I'm very depressed. Other times I am sort of sad."

"Are there things that seem to help?"

"Yes, it's best when other people are around and there are things to keep me busy."

"Does travelling help?"

"Yes, travelling is fine. Depression is a burden that I shall probably have to always struggle with."

"That may be true, but you can learn to deal with it."

"Right. You have to be optimistic."

"Absolutely. Another helpful thing, I find, is offering up my depression to God for all the suffering in the world."

"Yes, there are lots of unhappy adults and children who need assistance and prayers to help them through their miserable days," types Kevin.

"Does talking about it help?"

"Talking about my thoughts helps make my troubles lighter."

"Don't you like this music?"

"This is a sad song," Kevin writes concerning Rita McNeil's singing.

"Listening to sad songs can be entertaining."

"That may be true but I'm not in the mood today."

"When I was little, my mother would sing me sad songs and we'd both cry. We loved it. Don't you sometimes like sad songs?"

"Perhaps, but usually I don't like sad songs."

"Anyway, this is a plaintive love song that Rita wrote about the island that she loves."

"She wrote a beautiful tribute to Cape Breton. I like Rita McNeil and her music." A bit of background information goes a long way with Kevin.

"Now do you appreciate the song more?"

"Yes, I understand it better now."

At the Grassy Narrows exhibit, Kevin types, "That was interesting that the French attacked Grassy Narrows and they were allowed to keep Louisbourg."

"I wondered at that, too. No doubt there is an explanation."

Later in the day, we reach the Isaac's Harbour ferry crossing, and find the place deserted. "What a thing! To be stuck in no man's land with no ferry in sight," I joke.

"It's not very encouraging."

"It says they make additional crossings in an emergency. Maybe I should start screaming that I'm in pain."

"I think they'd be mad if you faked an emergency."

"Now that your mood has brightened with the sun, what per cent of the time do you think you're depressed?"

"About 40 per cent of the time." His estimate has not changed.

"Really?"

"Yes."

"What about when you're in school?"

"Especially when I'm in school."

"Why?"

"I know I could be doing much better but I can't communicate my knowledge."

"I hope you do well in school in September because this is your last semester and you will have a high school certificate."

"I hope so, but I will need a facilitator."

"The St. Francis House people will try to supply one."

"Why can't you be?" asks Kevin.

"I have to work."

"Why can't you take some time off work to come across to the school?" St. Joseph's Health Centre, where I work, is across the street from St. Pat's High School.

"It's a thought," I say. "Maybe I should do that instead of going to the seminary the first semester."

"Then for sure I would always say the right things." Apparently Kevin doesn't think he always said the "right things" with his other facilitators.

"If I should do such a drastic thing, I would need a guarantee of excellent behaviour from you."

"Yes. I would behave very well."

In the late afternoon, we have a cigarette butt incident. As always, I am upset. "How could you eat such a disgusting thing?" I demand. "It would make me vomit."

"You must have a sensitive taste."

Soon we stop for the night at a collection of small, simple cabins in Sherbrooke. "What do you think of this cabin?" I ask, curious to hear Kevin's reaction.

"It's very primitive."

"Has it any merit?"

"Yes. It's peaceful and calm," he says.

"It has no TV," I point out.

"That's not a problem," Kevin says. "I will, as far as I can tell, sit and play with my corn." (For years, Kevin always carried a handful of dried beans, corn or pebbles in a small container or his pocket. He would sift them to calm himself. He still does this occasionally.)

"Will you be able to settle down for bed?"

"Yes. I will settle down after I have something to eat."

### 1988 – Year of promise for St. Francis Advocates

In September 1988, a year after Kevin returned home from Toronto, we received confirmation from the Ministry of Community and Social Services that, under the joint Ministries of Housing and Social Services Project 3000, the operating monies for the project had been secured.[1]

Revenue Canada requested a financial statement and proof of our activities. In response, we proudly pointed out to Revenue Canada that our expertise would be in four areas. First, we would provide *housing* for adults exhibiting symptoms of autism. The setting would emphasize ongoing education and the acquisition and practice of communication and social skills, as well as independence. St. Francis Advocates would attend to the emotional, spiritual and physical needs of each individual, respecting persons of every race and creed.

Second, we would remain involved in *research* on autism. Third, we would continue in a *liaison* capacity between clients in institutions and their families, as well as between clients/families and ministries/agencies. Lastly, we would be a *resource* on autism and communication disabilities. To this end, we were already building a library of books, videos and other materials, and giving presentations to students and community groups.

Finally, in late April, the letter we had been awaiting arrived! The Ministry of Community and Social Services informed us that it was "pleased to advise that your project has been approved in principle to receive operating support funding from this Ministry."

But it was not until September that we received confirmation that, under the joint ministries of Health and Social Services Project 3000, "the operating monies for this project have been secured."

To facilitate proceedings from this point forward, the board hired a program director, Arden Stanlake.

### 1989 – St. Francis House opens

In October 1989, St. Francis House, a peaceful 25-acre hobby farm situated five miles southeast of Petrolia, opened its doors. Establishing it had taken eight years of personal time and five years of persistence by dedicated St. Francis Advocates.

The house is spacious, with private rooms for each of its five tenants, one of whom was Kevin. The occupants came from Petrolia, Chatham and Guelph; one came from the Southwestern Regional Centre in Dealtown. Regular family contact and home visits were encouraged as an integral part of the St. Francis Advocates' philosophy.

At this unofficial opening, the St. Anthony Fraternity of the Secular Franciscans presented a plaque with the Prayer of St. Francis and the San Damiano Cross.

Ten full-time staff and several part-time ones were needed to provide round-the-clock supervision. Elizabeth Blair, Assistant Program Director, and Karen Kelders, House Manager, assisted Arden Stanlake.

"High functioning teenagers and adults with autism need a 'mentor' to help them develop their interests, assist them with social skills, and motivate them to succeed," writes Dr. Temple Grandin.[2] The St. Francis Advocates board was optimistic that it had found several such mentors.

### Longing to be loved

As St. Francis Advocates opened its first residence, the board and staff were still developing policies and procedures. The process included examining policies from established group homes and making alterations as desired. Not surprisingly, a policy to deal with sexual behaviours and sex education for vulnerable adults proved the most difficult to formulate.

The policy models we examined pointed out that sexual expression could include a wide range of physical activities and the use of sexual aids. Heterosexual and homosexual intimacy between "consenting adults" was to be encouraged as a right. Those people choosing to abstain from sexual activity were to have this choice respected, but with the understanding that their choice could change over time.

Having pornography in one's own room should be a personal choice, many policies noted. Several programs included the recommendation of teaching masturbation to any developmentally delayed client whose agitated behaviours could *presumably* be caused by sexual tension.

Seeking further enlightenment, two of us from the St. Francis Advocates Board attended a workshop in London on "Sex Education for the Mentally Handicapped." There we were shown a video demonstrating how to teach masturbation. We were disturbed and puzzled. This was not at all what we wanted for any of our sons and daughters in or out of residential care.

Granted, the St. Francis Advocates' admission policy stated that we welcomed persons of every race, religion and ethnic origin. But we could not believe that our Christian values would clash with any of these regarding respect for human dignity. Indeed, parents seeking admission for their sons and daughters often expressed concern for the physical well-being of their children. Some cited past incidents of sexual abuse that they hoped would never be repeated.

Following much deliberation, the board and management of St. Francis Advocates came up with an interim policy stating that parents would be consulted should any sexual issue arise.

In the early 1990s, while studying at St. Peter's Seminary in London, I had the good fortune to take several courses from ethics author and professor, Father Michael Prieur. Under his mentoring I created a program in spirituality and sexuality for persons with developmental challenges. Field education projects were accepted at the seminary in lieu of theses, and this project became my final unit.

It was a major undertaking, but the timing of the program was providential. Kevin had begun challenging me about lapses in his education regarding sexuality. In the spring of 1992, he said, "You should understand that I have feelings, and you should help me deal with them."

"What can I do?" I asked.

"You should talk to me about special things like sexual feelings."

Shortly after that conversation, an article on autism appeared in a local paper. "That was a nice article in the paper, Kevin," I commented. "What did you think of it?"

"Perhaps it could have been better."

"Why is that?"

"It forgot to say people with autism perhaps have thoughts and feelings," said Kevin. "Perhaps we should write something else for the paper."

When I asked Kevin what he thought should be included in an article, he had an immediate response. "I want people to know we have normal thoughts and feelings." He again insisted that people with developmental delays should have courses in sexuality. "We should be told things that other people know and then we will not make fools of ourselves," he added. Kevin was alluding to a staff incident the preceding week where he had been taken to task for typing crude sexual comments to a female counsellor. He pleaded that he thought that was how you told someone you liked her.

A few weeks later, Kevin and I were watching a popular television sitcom. "Why are the Commish and his wife talking about abortion?" asked Kevin.

"They're afraid their baby might be handicapped."

"But wouldn't that make it dead?"

"Yes."

"That's terrible. Handicapped people are as important as people who are normal."

"Absolutely," I agreed. "All people should be treated with respect and love."

"And after handicapped people die, they go to God and then they're not handicapped anymore."

I was humbled by my son's innate wisdom, and thought of my own upcoming spirituality-sexuality program. "When I teach my course in the fall, do you think I will have to simplify things?" I asked.

"No, you should talk to them just like you talk to me. They're smarter than you think. Don't you realize they are all autistic and understand more than you realize? They're locked in the prisons of their bodies and their bizarre behaviours."

The program took place over a twelve-week period with the assistance of a fellow parishioner, Ray Chalmers. It was open to persons with disabilities throughout the county, their families, friends, and residential staff. We invited community agencies to share their resources and expertise with us.

A social worker from the Family Counselling Centre used excellent slides and posters in his anatomy session. Right to Life had realistic models of developing foetuses that participants were delighted to hold and examine in their hands. The sexual assault coordinator from my hospital shared important information on the safety of vulnerable populations. Father Pricur gave two inspiring presentations on discipleship and sexual ethics: one to our class, and a second to a larger, community-wide audience.

For reasons of consistency and complexity, we chose not to address issues of contraception or sexual preferences in our program. I remember one young woman taking me aside and whispering that she had a secret: her uterus had been removed. "I don't have periods, and I can't have babies," she explained. I vaguely remember thanking her for sharing her secret with me. I also remember thinking it was less complicated to have a son. Parents and individuals have various situations to deal with. Each deserves consideration and a thoughtful approach. Each individual deserves to be treated respectfully, to receive ongoing education, to participate in personal decisions, and to be aided in developing an informed conscience.

According to Thomas and Donna Finn, an informed conscience understands that the way we treat one another sexually has a lasting impact on our innermost sense of who we are. It is one which is open to pursuing the knowledge of a true right and a true wrong. It starts with an open question, and seeks information on all sides of the subject – not as a means of confirming one's bias or defensively held opinion, but rather as a means of determining the truth concerning the issue at hand, much like a courtroom jury is called upon to do.[3]

Since the time of those presentations, I have contemplated the many controversies surrounding sexuality in modern life, and its implications for developmentally delayed people. We consider the past to have been overly rigid in its attitudes towards sexuality, but the present would seem far too lenient.

Jean Vanier looks at one example of changed social attitudes.

> In the past, masturbation was rigidly condemned. This condemnation led to fear, which nourished guilt and led to inhibitions, even hatred of oneself and one's body. Today, there is a tendency to say that masturbation is not serious, that we should let people do what they want, and that it is normal for an adolescent. It seems to me that the truth is between these two attitudes of rigidity and permissiveness. One must not condemn young people who masturbate. They have compulsions which they are not yet able to control or integrate. However, it is necessary to help them to stop. Masturbation can close them in on themselves and into a world of dreams and thus prevent them from entering into true relationships.[4]

How do we find true relationships for ourselves, and how can we assist those who have developmental and emotional delays? Kevin and I have touched upon this topic in several of our conversations.

"About people not getting married until they can be independent, perhaps I will never be independent," he commented one day.

I replied that being responsible is more important than being independent. "Some people who always need assistance do get married," I said.

"What do you mean by responsible?" asked Kevin.

"Responsible is being able to make sensible decisions and having a certain amount of maturity," I replied. "Everything in life takes practice."

"I'm not perhaps able to be a good husband. But I want to practice learning how to act mature."

On another occasion, Kevin told me, "I'm not sure that I will ever get married."

"How do you feel about that?" I asked.

"As far as I know, that will be fine. I will still have family and friends and God."

Kevin understands that we are created to be in relationship whether we are married or single. But, contrary to modern cultural imagery, all genuine human relationships call for chastity. In the married life, chastity calls us to a relationship that is permanent, exclusive and honest. In the single state, chastity invites warm, loving relationships that exclude sexual intercourse.

A person can live a chaste life whether they be heterosexual or homosexual. Each is very much a child of God with great value and dignity of personhood. Each must develop a strong prayer life and personal relationships with others in order to lead a happy, fulfilled life.

Temple Grandin, a professor and animal behaviour expert who is herself autistic, says that "many people with autism avoid complicated sex issues by remaining celibate. Celibacy is the course I have taken. My career is exciting and my life is my work."[5] Grandin has the emotional maturity to be comfortable with her lifestyle decisions.

Those who have not yet developed this level of maturity look to available role models for their choices. A vulnerable person may be at the level of "self-centredness and pervasive sense of inadequacy" combined with an "acute sense of not belonging" typical of adolescence. It has been found that sexual permissiveness leads to "empty relationships, feelings of self-contempt and worthlessness." A study of college students showed that, although their sexual behaviour "appeared to be a desperate attempt to overcome a profound sense of loneliness, they described their sexual relationships as less than satisfactory and as providing little of the emotional closeness they desired. Moreover, they described pervasive feelings of guilt and haunting concerns that they were using others and being used as sexual objects."[6]

With today's society fixated on sexual fantasy, sexual preoccupation and superficial relationships, the media in all its forms promotes questionable models. Everywhere we look, we are told that we should expect love and admiration without assuming responsibility. And thus the most vulnerable are encouraged to remain forever emotionally immature. Adolescent fixations and emotional immaturity cannot lead to solid relationships. In seeking personal relationships, we want these to be authentic friendships based on trust and respect. Author Ann Bouchard writes that her own criterion for genuine friendship is

> faithfulness: that is, the friendship helps and supports my friend to be faithful in keeping his or her commitments, and me in keeping mine. While remaining faithful, one stands by the other in joy and sorrow. In that criterion is ample room for dying to oneself and living for others, not trying to possess the other, staying free and leaving free.[7]

Human sexuality is the energy behind creativity, relationship and love. Sexual energy, the very energy through which God created the universe, is integral to our beings. "There is, in the sexual attraction, the simple cry of a body longing to be loved and touched with tenderness by another," says Jean Vanier.[8]

Longing to be loved. This cry for relationship is embedded in our humanity. However, as Father Raymond Dlugos of the Southdown Institute, a treatment centre for clergy, pointed out at a recent workshop, "in its most creative and energizing form, sexual energy requires boundaries."[9]

Freedom and boundaries complement each other. It's because we have boundaries that we enjoy freedom in our land and within our lives. Uncontrolled sexuality as portrayed by movies and media is merely power, domination and exploitation. The "best point of departure is conservative, because first you need a clear feeling for your own boundaries," agrees Richard Rohr. The more you become sure of your own centre, the more you can open your boundaries. Otherwise you'll spend your whole life defending those boundaries, which is an indication of immaturity. "Nevertheless," says Rohr, "we have to be patient and allow ourselves to take certain steps toward growth. A mature Christian is capable of going beyond all previous boundaries and suddenly discovering Christ where he or she would never have suspected."[10]

When we discuss sexuality and relationships with persons who have limitations of mind, body or maturity, we must do so honestly, yet sensitively. It is not useful, kind or respectful to make light of an individual's longing for companionship. It is to be hoped that there *will* be a special person or persons in his or her life.

And what about the claim that sexuality is our own business, a private affair? Henri Nouwen has some thoughts on this subject.

> Sexual fantasies, sexual thoughts, sexual actions are mostly seen as belonging to the private life of a person. But the distinction between the private and the public sphere of life is a false distinction and has created many of the problems we are struggling with in our day. In the Christian life the distinction between a private life (just for me!) and a public life (for the others) does not exist.[11]

The mental and spiritual health of a society is dependent on the way its members live their most personal lives as a service to their fellow human beings. Regardless of the extent of our vulnerabilities, we are called to lives of integrity within the boundaries we have chosen. In teaching those with limitations to live within boundaries, we are offering them peace of mind and freedom of heart.

### Spiritual journey

Sexuality is the longing within us for connection, the life force that makes us interested in others. Without sexuality, we would choose solitude over community. God created us for relationships, and Jesus tells us to love one another as he has loved us.

Although some people with disabilities may feel they have no choice in their celibate-by-necessity lifestyle, they can learn from those whose vocation includes celibacy freely chosen. Franciscans Murray Bodo and Frances Teresa tell us that just as sexual activity does not necessarily include intimacy, so intimacy need not include sexual activity.

"What intimacy does include," says Bodo, "is our sexuality itself, our maleness and/or femaleness. We love God and people as men and women, not as sexless automatons. And the only restrictions to our loving are God's command to love him and our neighbour as ourselves and the promises we have made to him and/or another human being. Common sense and our own good heart usually supply the rest."[12]

Sister Frances Teresa points out that Francis and Clare "became exemplars of the rich possibilities latent in celibacy which, to be fruitful, must have a focus beyond itself on which we can concentrate our energies. No one will be fruitfully celibate if their celibacy is rooted in a refusal of intimacy, a rejection of human needs or a denial of sexuality."[13] We are called to reveal God to each other in our mutual courtesy, love and respect for one another.

I asked Kevin's brothers and father what kind of relationships, including sexual, persons with developmental disabilities should have. They admitted to struggling with their responses, but nonetheless wrote down their thoughts.

> I believe that persons have the right to a relationship that they are mentally and emotionally able to deal with [says James]. In addition, with proper guidance and education, developmentally disabled persons have the right to sexual relationships provided they are able to effectively deal with the possible outcomes, including the ability to care for children. I also believe that in some cases, unfortunately, developmentally disabled persons will simply be unable to form healthy relationships (especially sexual relationships). Furthermore, in some cases, the state may in fact need to step in to protect one or both individuals (and any children that

could result). It would be a vast understatement to say that these interventions will not be easy for society to make.

I am convinced that Kevin will have many positive relationships and friendships in his lifetime. It is also my opinion, however, that Kevin is unable to deal with a sexual relationship (or its possible outcomes) at this time.

I struggle with the complexity of the issues in relationships [says Chris]. Of course, relationships can be intricate, especially sexual relationships. From a religious standpoint, people should be married when engaging in a sexual relationship. But would we encourage marriage? Who would decide if people with developmental disabilities are capable of marriage? Is it really anyone's business to decide? Do we have an obligation to discourage a marriage if it is obvious that the two individuals are not capable of existing in a marriage? Who would decide? What right does society have to decide? What rights do individuals have to decide on their own?

Consider sexual relationships outside of marriage. Should it be discouraged? What about two consenting developmentally disabled adults? Could you physically stop them? Consider birth control. The Church is against it. Should people with developmental disabilities be educated regarding birth control? Should they be encouraged to use it? Should they be forced to use it? Should they be forced not to use it? What if they wanted to get pregnant? What would happen if a pregnancy resulted? Would society allow them to raise their own child? Should they be allowed to raise a child? There are so many questions that it boggles the mind. Regarding Kevin, I am under the impression that having such relationships is not an interest of his. If he was interested, I feel he should be provided with all possible information.

With the proper teaching [says Joel], and as long as it's with the right person, relationships can be the same for persons with disabilities as with anyone else. We are all entitled to love and be loved. With sexuality, I feel the person should clearly be aware, or be made aware of, the difference between lust and love. With Kevin, it would be the same, but I guess I would want to be ensured that both parties are fully understanding of the situation.

While working in the social field, I often became frustrated when people were perfectly fine with the individuals acting promiscuously with each other. They would say, "They're adults; they can do what they want." However, I felt that was way too simple. Other questions needed to be asked, such as Is it consensual? Are the persons aware of all the options, such as other relationships? Are they aware of the consequences, both emotionally and physically? Are they simply bored? All these questions should definitely be asked of Kevin for any of his future relationships.

Says Jim, "If there's a problem, handle it with individual counselling. I think many group home policies assume there has to be a problem where there may not be."

And what does Kevin now think? "There is too much emphasis on sex instead of sexuality, which is the creative essence of our beings," he says. "We are meant to live in respectful, loving relationships in our families and other communities." Kevin's ideal is, in fact, the one held by Francis and Clare in their love towards each other, and for the companions of their shared vision.

Franciscans see work as a partnership with God's creative power, forever active in our world.

# 7

# Hope and Dreams

**From Kevin's journal: Days 13 and 14**

*Day 13 — July 29, 1992 — Halifax*

"Are we leaving Nova Scotia?" asks Kevin anxiously.

"Not for four or five days," I reassure him.

"Good. I like it here."

"Are you feeling more cheerful today?"

"As far as I can tell, better than yesterday, but still a bit sad."

Some time later, Kevin becomes agitated. "Don't go back to Ecum Secum," he insists. "It's not important to me to have my picture taken there. I would rather have my picture taken at West Quoddy."

"You seem to be angry about something," I note.

"Yes. I'm angry because Dad likes Ecum Secum."

"Dad is entitled to his likes and dislikes. If he likes Ecum Secum, we should humour him."

"Yes. You're right," he admits.

Later, at the Bedford Institute of Oceanography, Kevin types, "I'm bored."

"How do you know you will not act this way at school?"

"As far as I can tell, I have to study hard."

"It may seem boring."

"I will behave."

"I want a beer shirt," he tells us later when we stop in at the Moosehead Beer Factory to inquire about tours.

"You do?" I ask.

"Yes."

"What colour?"

"Green."

After considerable discussion on places to eat in Halifax, we ask Kevin if he has a preference. "Let's go anywhere," he says. "I'm hungry."

"Dad likes to plan carefully but he thinks I'm impetuous. Do you know what impetuous means?"

"Snap decisions."

"Do you agree?"

"Yes, I do. And you have perhaps a quick temper."

"Kevin!" I say in mock horror.

As we drive away after dinner, Kevin is unable to locate his Memo Writer and we fear it has been left at the restaurant. We stop the car at Halifax Harbour for a frantic search and are greatly relieved to find it among our belongings.

"Here's your computer. We didn't leave it in the restaurant after all," I say.

"I'm relieved," says a smiling Kevin. "I would be helpless without it."

"Why are you flapping your hands?" I ask at another stop. "People are looking at you."

"It helps me focus on things. It helps my vision especially, but it also focuses my thoughts."

We shout at Kevin as he goes for his second butt of the day. He stops this time and asks, "Why should I not eat butts?"

"You tell *me*. List some reasons for not eating butts."

"Contamination. Disease. Poison my body. Look stupid. No coffee. It's an addiction."

"That's a very good list. You have an excellent mind, so use it."

Kevin collects travel pins. In one store I ask him, "What does this pin say on it?"

"Bluenose," he answers.

"Does that have any significance?"

"That's the boat we saw tonight."

*Day 14 – July 30, 1992 – Halifax, Dartmouth, Shelbourne*

"Quite a selection of very nice food, for a base. Why did we come here?" asks Kevin of Base Dartmouth.

"Because it's interesting and inexpensive."

"Where are we going today?"

"We have laundry to do and shopping in a mall. Does this base have any significance?"

"James came here to do officer training."

"How do you know that?"

"I heard you and Dad talking yesterday."

Later, Kevin inquires, "What are you and Dad talking about?"

"We're talking about your last semester of school, when you'll be doing proper courses."

"As far as I can tell, I will need your help."

"You'll be doing history and English and possibly math."

"I hardly know a thing about math but I would like to learn."

In the laundromat, Kevin becomes annoyed. "Why are you angry?" I ask.

"I'm angry that you are doing laundry."

"Everybody who wears clothing has to do laundry. Do you want to go shopping with Dad while I stay here?"

"Yes. That's fine."

"Will you avoid butts?"

"Yes, if Dad reminds me at each stop."

But Jim and Kevin return with an all-too-common negative report. "Kevin, why did you eat a butt?" I sigh.

"I wanted to be bad. Today is boring."

"What were you thinking when you ate the butt?"

"I don't know why I did that. I feel unhappy with myself and I want everybody else to be unhappy, too."

"I'm reading about that very thing," I say. "Read this paragraph and tell me what you read."

"It says that it's easy to escape into the pleasure of drugs," says Kevin after reading. "But the person needs to be helped. They need to grow towards life, not death."

"And what can help?"

"Patience and prayer."

"Dad still wants to know why you ate that butt."

"I was being mean to him because I felt little. He treated me in an immature way. He told me to be a good boy and I am a man."

"When you conquer your addictions, you will be free and healthy and happier," I tell my son.

"I want you to help me grow healthy. I will try harder. I want to be normal. I want to be happier. I will pray and study and talk out my problems."

"Why are you angry?" I ask. Kevin is saying the right words, but his body language is not in agreement.

"I'm angry that you're telling me I have to help myself."

"But you most certainly must."

"When are we going west?" It is amazing how abruptly Kevin can proceed to an unrelated topic in the midst of an angry tirade.

"We're in no hurry. Do you want to tour the Moosehead Beer Factory?"

"Yes. That would be interesting. When are we going there?"

"Tomorrow morning."

When we stop for a rest, Kevin and his father have a conversation. "Why do you have a problem carrying out instructions sometimes?" asks Jim.

"I get confused when I have to do something."

"Can you explain it?"

"As far as I can tell, it has to do with motor activity," says Kevin.

"Do you seem to get stuck?'

"Yes, I often seem to get stuck when I have to move, and I can't get started."

"How can we help?" asks his father.

"You can tell me to start."

"But that doesn't always help," points out Jim.

"As far as I can tell, you have to wait a bit and then I do it. You are sometimes too impatient and then I get more stuck."

"It's difficult for me to tell if you're stuck or simply refusing to do something," says Jim.

"That is because I seem to be defiant and am being rebellious," replies Kevin.

"And why would you be defiant and rebellious?"

"That's one of the few controls I have in my life."

"Kevin, quit jumping around," I say, as we walk along. "What do people think when you do that?"

"They would think I didn't understand."

"They'd have no idea how clever you are."

In our motel room that evening, I ask Kevin, "How are you tonight?"

"I'm fine."

"And how is our holiday?"

"It's good. Where are we going tomorrow?"

"We're going to travel around the south coast of Nova Scotia and see some beautiful places, like Peggy's Cove."

"That's great."

"Anything of note on the news?" I ask, testing his powers of observation.

"It's perhaps exciting that Canada won a gold [medal]. You should give me supper."

"You poor, neglected waif."

"Yes, I am a neglected waif."

"But do you feel loved?"

"Yes. I'm deeply loved by my family."

"You certainly are."

"We are happier than most families."

"Do you think it's right that we withhold coffee when you eat butts?"

"It's perhaps not fair because I can't help myself."

"But your counsellor doesn't want you eating butts."

"It's true she doesn't want me eating butts," says Kevin. "However, she does not feel I should be punished."

"So what should we do when you eat butts?"

"You should be nice to me if I eat butts."

"And that will help you quit eating butts?" I ask.

"Yes."

We also talk about Kevin's future. "Everyone has to have a dream," I say, "so that they have a path to follow. What's your dream?"

"I want to be independent and have a university degree," says Kevin. "Then I can advocate for social justice for the handicapped."

"What subjects do you want to study in university?"

"English, religion and psychology."

"That sounds like a good choice."

## The inner vision

Hope and dreams are lifetime gifts infused in our beings by God, the Creator of all things. Hope adds sparkle to our lives, and dreams motivate us to move forward creatively. Both are powerful gifts, enriching our souls and enhancing the way we think and act.

Small children already have their heroes and can tell us what they want to become. A firefighter! A police officer! A doctor! Their faces light up when they tell us these things.

When I was young, one of the careers I considered was truck driving. Since I loved travelling, it seemed to me that being paid to drive all over Canada and the United States would be the ideal career choice. I do not recall discussing this with my parents or teachers, but I carried within me the confidence that I could accomplish anything I set out to do. The adults in my life made me feel valued and important. I always had an abundance of hope and a profusion of dreams.

Throughout our lives, hope keeps us on course. St. Paul calls hope "a sure and steadfast anchor of the soul" (Hebrews 6:19). Then faith, that precious gift of God, gives promise to our hope. Faith is "the assurance of things hoped for, the conviction of things not seen" (Hebrews 11:1). Paul tells us that we must first have hope for faith to take root. The anchor of hope grounds us, stilling our souls so that we can serenely proceed in our faith journey.

Dreams evolve and change, but they lead us forward like beacons. The mundane parts of our days are flavoured by our dreams. A person on an assembly line may amuse himself with the thought of his fishing trip two weekends away. A doctor, seeing patient after endless patient on a long and tiring day, looks forward to the plans she has made for her day off. Of course, we also have larger long-term dreams that pull us towards career goals and influence decisions regarding family, social justice or vocational choices.

Kevin and his housemates, Dave and Dave, look forward to bowling, movies, concerts at Hiawatha Raceway, and other recreational events. This seems to shorten the time they spend folding laundry at the nursing home where they work.

"Dave and Dave are my good friends," Kevin told me recently, "and we do lots of neat things together. I hope that, as we get older, we can still have holidays together and do some travelling. Maybe we can sometimes travel with you and Dad."

"Where would you like to travel?"

"Anywhere, as long as it's a long trip."

"Do you have some favourite places?"

"I love Nova Scotia. Europe was wonderful, too. Probably my most favourite place in the world is Assisi. It was so peaceful and beautiful there, and I felt so close to God, especially at San Damiano."

Dreams change as our lives proceed, and hope carries us from one dream to the next. Human limitations influence the process. When we were younger, Jim and I thrived on long, adventurous trips. We thought nothing of travelling 500 miles in a day, eager to see as much of North America as we possibly could in the time available to us. Pulling our tent trailer behind our van crammed with children, pets and camping paraphernalia, we travelled far from home, sharing the roadways and camps with the roving hippies and flower children of the 1960s and '70s. Even in the following two decades, we managed one long trip a year.

But lately Jim and I have developed a preference for shorter trips with longer stretches of staying in place. Whenever time permits, we park our motor home amidst the trees of Pinery Provincial Park. There we choose the shadiest, most private locations where Jim can read, and I can write and daydream, while our pets lie lazily about. Kevin is often with us, enjoying hikes and campfires.

Anticipating our next camping experience is one of the dreams that floats us through the in-between times of work, committee meetings and community activities.

What we do with our lives is shaped by many factors. Limitations of mind and body certainly play a role. But more important are life experiences, encouragement and opportunities.

Kevin would like to interact more meaningfully with the world around him. From time to time, he longs for a career that will free him from the monotony of his laundry job. Not long ago, he told us that he thought he would like to be a nature photographer. "That would perhaps be easier than writing," he suggested. He also hoped that learning photography "would be a way of reaching out to the world." We gave him some disposable cameras to practise on. Since then, he has concluded, possibly realistically, that he doesn't think he has sufficient physical dexterity to operate photographic equipment.

Writing is something that has always appealed to Kevin because he feels he has worthwhile things to say. After completing high school, he began a correspondence course in journalism. He tried very hard, but found it to be too much work and very tiring. Keeping focused through the labyrinth of autistic brain functioning is undoubtedly an exhausting experience.

At the time, Kevin expressed the belief that staff members at the farm residence were "too stressed to help me." Certainly, I myself found that helping him with his correspondence homework on weekends was laborious. I admired the staff for their effort. Writing is a time-consuming process for any author. When the process is complicated by the necessity of facilitated communication, it can become frustrating for both author and assistant. Certainly, it can't help but take away much of the spontaneity necessary in any creative venture.

A more rewarding experience for Kevin took place when he accompanied me to St. Peter's Seminary during the 1993–94 academic year, auditing two classes. "I loved the seminary," Kevin said. "It was so exciting to be there with all the seminarians and priests and students. They treated me like I was another student, and they valued me. I hated to see the year come to an end. I loved the atmosphere and the beautiful buildings and chapel. I became an important man for once in my life."

Our days are motivated by goals that change over time. When disabled people seem to have unrealistic hopes and dreams, rather than discourage them, we can inspire them by encouraging them to proceed with the early steps towards their goal. Who really knows how far any one of us will get?

Hope and dreams can be stifled and fade away. Since the world began, people young and old, with and without limitations, lose hope and have their dreams smothered by their environment. The prophet Daniel wrote that the people who were with him did not see his vision, "though a great trembling fell upon them, and they fled and hid themselves. So I was left alone to see this great vision" (Daniel 10:7-8).

Temple Grandin describes how the encouragement of others freed her to use her superior visualization skills, despite the severe deficits caused by autism. Speaking of her ease at drawing elaborate images of livestock stockyards, she says she is "able to visualize a motion picture of the finished facility in my imagination. When I was a child, my parents and teachers recognized my artistic talents. Talents need to be nurtured and developed."[1]

When those we love are challenged by limitations, we are called upon to keep their hope alive by believing in their dreams. Kevin's dream of being a writer is being accomplished in this book, which he is co-authoring with me. We believe in his capability, and will help him keep his dream alive in the coming years. There are other writing projects under consideration that we can do together. Perhaps Kevin will find a faithful assistant, such as Helen Keller had. With God's help, Kevin will continue to work towards the independence of his hopes and dreams.

## Spiritual journey

Our purpose in life is to give others hope: hope that God is always in our midst, hope that God is within each person and reaches out to us through those we encounter in our life activities. Parents and teachers consider it their responsibility and vocation to impart motivation and inspiration. Clare of Assisi saw it as her "primary vocation – to reveal God, reflect God's light and glory."[2]

While experiencing the abject misery of life in a Nazi concentration camp, professor and psychotherapist Viktor Frankl was able to visualize his suffering as if viewing it from the safety of the future. He could see himself in a warm lecture hall "giving a lecture on the psychology of the concentration camp."[3] Frankl taught fellow prisoners this visualizing technique as a method of escape through dreams.

Kevin continues to hope for and dream of a more independent future. Recently he told me that if he had his own money he would be "able to do what I want with my life and be able to have some say in my life. I would work at doing interesting things like gardening and reading and travelling."

"What about Fiddick's [the nursing home where Kevin works]?" I asked.

"I would work at Fiddick's one or two days a week and have an assistant for other times."

"Where would you live?" I wondered.

"I would perhaps live half-time with the Daves and half-time with you, and my assistant would follow me."

"Would you want your assistant to be a man or a woman, and how old should that person be?"

"I think it should be a man, but a woman might be okay. The assistant should be my age."

Before my association with people who cannot deny their limitations, I would not have looked to them for inspiration. But vulnerable persons, and their less vulnerable companions, have taught me the art of mutuality. In their company, I have received genuine empathy, affection, and encouragement. How can one not return such generosity?

In an earlier age, Francis of Assisi discovered the contagious power of the joy of humble persons. "Indeed, whenever I am tempted or depressed," Francis observed, "if I see my companions joyful, I immediately turn away from my temptation and oppression, and regain my own inward and outward joy."[4]

The tragedy in our world is not that some people have disabilities — we all do! — but that these people are not given encouragement and opportunities to use their gifts. We enrich *ourselves* when we help release these gifts. Drawing on personal experience to describe a family's walk with autism, V.C. Keating writes of the positive nature of hope and dreams:

> We are still walking through the maze but flowers bloom beside the road. A warm, gentle wind tousles our hair and teases our senses with floral fragrance.
>
> We stop to enjoy the song of a bird, and suddenly hundreds and thousands of bird voices create a chorus of trills and warbles. The music expands in timbre and density until it seems that a celestial choir has exploded in melodious sound, which drifts to us from distant peaks and blends with nature here below.[5]

Lately, Kevin has been excited about helping me edit the newsletter for St. Francis Advocates. He already has some ideas for it. "It should have information about all the people, and each issue should focus on one house or group. It should have interviews with the people, and I could ask them questions." This will be a new undertaking for both of us – another dream brought to life by the energy of hope.

Both hope, which provides confidence, and dreams, which motivate us to embrace creation, are fed from the life-giving springs of grace within us. Indeed, Jesus tells us that "the kingdom of God is within" us (Luke 17:21). Carrying the divine kingdom within us as we go about our lives, accompanied by the communion of saints, we cannot help but be inspired. It is no wonder that our hopes and dreams are powerfully persuasive.

All vulnerable to one degree or another, we are rightful members of God's kingdom and worthy companions of the communion of saints. Everyone, vulnerable and less so, needs reminders to activate their marvellous spiritual gifts through prayer. Communicating with God alters our lives. "As we dive deeper into God's presence, we divest ourselves of what is superfluous," says Patti Normile. "Unnecessary attitudes, worries, fear and angers float to the surface to be carried away by God's loving care. What we discover, as Francis realized, is that God is not in the trappings in which we have enshrined God, but within us."[6]

When we make this same discovery, we become truly aware of our power and gifts. We acquire the inspiration to don the armour of hope and the courage to follow our dreams. Moreover, we recognize that our brothers and sisters rely on our prayerful intervention. The efficacy of intercessory prayer has long been recognized. Charles Theisler cites a controlled study where, unknown to the patients themselves, various religious groups prayed for hospitalized coronary patients. "In comparing outcomes between the test and control groups it was found that the recipients of prayer fared much better," Theisler says. "The group receiving prayer had significantly lower severity scores. The prayer group required less ventilatory assistance, fewer antibiotics and diuretics than control groups."[7]

Prayer and contemplation are the essence of Franciscan spirituality, the soul of all we are and do. "Let them participate in the sacramental life of the Church," instructs the Rule, "above all the Eucharist. Let them join in liturgical prayer in one of the forms proposed by the Church, reliving the mysteries of the life of Christ."[8]

Like all Franciscans, those of the Secular Order follow the example of Francis of Assisi, "who made Christ the inspiration and the centre of his life with God and people."[9] By revealing God to the vulnerable in their midst, Francis and Clare freed the broken spirits of their humble brothers and sisters. In making Jesus the centre of our lives, we are called to encourage the vulnerable to soar with their hopes and dreams.

# 8

# Limitations

**From Kevin's journal: Days 15 and 16**

*Day 15 – July 31, 1992 – Shelbourne*

"You're so grouchy today, Kev," I observe. "What are you grumpy about?"

"I'm upset because I have to go back to St. Francis House."

"But you'll be going back to life, your future, your studies – all the exciting things that are waiting to happen. Holidays are to rest us up so we can tackle another chunk of life."

"I'm glad to hear that."

"Do you feel better?'

"Yes."

But later in the morning, there is another outburst. "Now what?" I ask.

"I'm angry that we're not going on the beer factory tour."

"We *are* going on the tour. What made you think we weren't?"

"You said we were going to the mall."

"First we're going to the mall to pick up my top that's being altered."

"Okay."

"Think of something to be happy about."

"I'm happy we have perhaps a week left of our holidays," says Kevin.

"And what can you look forward to?" I prompt.

"As far as I can tell, I can look forward to classes in September."

"Right! And also, you're still going on holidays with St. Francis House."

"When are you going on holidays with them?" asks his dad.

"As far as I can tell, we will be going on holidays on the 15th so I will not be home for two weeks."

"That should be nice," I say.

"Yes, because I've had all this time with you. I'm looking forward to you facilitating for me in school."

"We'll have to have a planning meeting about that."

"Yes, you'll have to meet with Arden and the teachers."

"What do you expect to see in the beer factory?" I ask Kevin now.

"I think they will show us how they brew the beer and then bottle it."

"I always knew that you were smart, didn't I?"

"Yes. You always had faith in me and that's what gave me courage."

In the brewery waiting room, we browse through magazines, waiting for the tour to begin. "Here's an article on clowns," I say. "You could be a clown, Kevin. Clowns do mime. Do you know what that is?"

"Mime is acting without talking. Yes, that would be perhaps something I could learn to do. Then I could visit hospitals and institutions, and cheer people up. As far as I can tell, I could be a career clown and writer."

"That's an excellent idea. Let's go. The tour is going to begin."

"Great."

"It will last about 40 minutes," I repeat for Kevin's benefit.

"That's good. They should be able to tell us lots of assorted information in that time."

As we watch a video, Kevin begins to flick his fingers, making a clicking sound. "Quit all that flicking and try to look normal," I say. "Why are you so agitated?"

"Why do you care if I look normal? I want to leave. It's only a video."

"The tour will follow the video."

During the guided tour, I ask Kevin, "Do you understand what it's all about?"

"Yes, I think I understand it all. It's quite interesting and I'm really glad we came."

"Does the flicking help your comprehension?"

"Yes. It helps me understand."

"And you don't understand as clearly if you don't flick?"

"Yes."

We finish the tour, leave the brewery, and then...another incident!

"Are you angry?" he asks.

"I certainly am," I say.

"I couldn't help it. You should try to understand."

"I have tried."

"Then try some more."

"You've eaten two butts this morning even though we gave you coffee after you ate the first one."

"I am upset. You were angry when I ate the other butt."

When next we facilitate, Kevin asks, "Are you still angry?"

"No. I'll keep trying to understand. Do you think we are making *any* progress in butts?"

"Yes. I'm less interested in their taste now. I'm more aware of the poison and disease."

At the Lunenburg Fisheries Museum, we ask Kevin which model of the Bluenose he wants.

"I like the big one attached to the plaque," he decides.

"What do you like about it?" I ask.

"I like it because it explains about the Bluenose. Are you still angry?"

"No."

We examine various fish in the museum's aquariums. Kevin types comments as we move from tank to tank. "I think they're ugly…it's even uglier than the lobster…I think these are gross…this is very ugly…the pout is ugly too…I like all these weird fish. Sculpin looks okay."

"What did that information on the lobster say?" I ask at one point.

"He weighs 15 pounds and is 25 years old from St. George Bay."

"St. George Banks."

"Right."

"Look at the haddock. They're a very tasty fish."

"They may taste good but they're ugly."

"Flounders are another type of flat fish."

"Flounders are strange," says Kevin.

"Look. What's that say?" I ask.

"Skate," Kevin replies, and then asks, "Why do the lobsters have their claws taped?"

"To prevent them from eating the other fish and cannibalizing each other."

"Why would they cannibalize each other?"

"They fight for territory when they are overcrowded."

"Do they do that in the ocean?" Kevin wonders.

"No, because they have space. Here is a blue lobster."

"Are they common?"

"The guide said one in a million."

"That's very rare."

"Do you understand *this* display, Kevin?" I ask.

"Yes. They close the net and pull it up."

"What's *he* doing?" I question, regarding a live demonstration by a fisherman.

"Giving a demonstration on filleting a fish. What is a parasite?"

"A worm that feeds on the fish."

"I'm glad they remove the parasites."

"When were we last on a ship?" asks Jim.

"At Mary's baptism two summers ago at Victoria," remembers Kevin. "This is very interesting. More interesting than the beer factory. I thought there would have been more to see there."

Before leaving, we buy Kevin the ship he had chosen earlier. "I'm happy that I have my nice Bluenose," he says with a smile.

"What will you do with it?"

"I want to take it home to St. Francis House and put it on the wall in my room."

"What have you liked best about our trip so far?"

"Seeing all the scenery. The lakes and forests and rocks and the ocean. It was very peaceful."

"There's a puzzle map of Canada. Do you understand it?"

"I know all about maps," Kevin said. In fact, we have learned that he knows far more than we had ever imagined.

*Day 16 – August 1, 1992 – Digby*

"How are you today, love?" I ask my son, following an evening and night when I had been incommunicado with a migraine.

"I'm fine and I'm glad you're feeling better. I hate it when you're sick."

"Why?" Undoubtedly, my migraines *have* had a negative impact on my family through the years. Although they have been severe and frequent, I tend to think they are limiting only to me. This is because I have been afflicted with the condition since the age of seven, and because I have rarely allowed it to keep me from work or routine activities. In hindsight, I have been medicated, dull, and withdrawn. Shrinking from light and noise, I am less than an exciting person to be around.

"We can enjoy ourselves more and eat real food," types Kevin.

"Real food?" I wonder.

"At a restaurant," replies Kevin.

I am wearing a green T-shirt bearing an autism logo. It occurs to me that Kevin may find it offensive. "How do you feel when I wear my autism T-shirt?" I ask.

"I like it because it tells people about autism," says Kevin. My son has a great attitude, and once again, I am filled with admiration.

During our next car trip, though, Kevin rocks in the back seat. When we stop, I ask him, "Were you angry?"

"Yes. I was angry about the rain."

"We can't do anything about the rain, and we've been very fortunate to have had wonderful weather all along."

"I guess so," admits Kevin.

Shortly afterwards, Kevin says, "Dad is silly today." He then says, "I was angry that I couldn't have coffee."

"That's unreasonable," I say. Kevin is unresponsive. "Aren't you going to answer?" I persist. "It's unreasonable because you've had four cups already today."

"You are bugging me. You're asking too many questions."

"Can't I tell you that you've had too much coffee?"

"No. I should be able to have as much coffee as I want."

"Actually, that's not correct. I'm not supposed to have more than two cups of coffee daily because of my migraines. People have to practice moderation in many ways for their health."

While travelling that day, we visit St. Mary's Church at Church Point. "Do you want to light a candle and pray for something special?" I ask.

"Yes. I want to pray that I will do well in school."

"What do you think?" I ask Kevin after he lights a candle from a wooden wick.

"It's a beautiful church and I liked lighting the prayer candle. I like the way it smells. It's almost as good as eating a butt."

Later we enjoy dinner in a Digby restaurant. "This is great," says Kevin. "I'm having haddock and baked potato. When are we going on the ferry?"

"Tomorrow."

"Where are we going?" he asks.

"To St. John, New Brunswick, and then to Maine for a few days."

"Great. As far as I can tell, we are having a good time in Nova Scotia."

Although we have asked Kevin this question before, Jim asks again for clarification, "What does that flicking do for you?"

"As far as I can tell, the flicking helps me to focus."

"And when you don't flick?" asks Jim.

"Then I'm less focused and I make mistakes."

"But don't you mind looking silly when you flick?" asks Jim.

"Quite an awful question. As far as I can tell, I can't control my hands and it's rude to stare."

Knowing I am a seafood person, Jim asks me if I would like lobster. I consider this, and ask Kevin the same question. "Would you like lobster for dinner?"

"Would it have to be killed?"

"Yes."

"How would they do it?"

"They boil them."

"Would it still be alive?"

"Yes, but they say they're in shock from the hot water and they die quickly."

"That is terrible. Quite cruel, I think," Kevin says.

"I'm having haddock," I decide, suddenly losing interest in lobster. "What do you want?"

"The same," says Kevin.

"What do you think of the wooden wick we bought for you?" asks Jim.

"Dad appears autistic when he sniffs that stick, and the thing is he can control himself. Therefore, quite unnecessary."

"You anticipated what I was going to say to *you*," says Jim.

"Quit teasing me. Quit being assertive. You are picking on me today and I have not done anything to you."

"Why is Dad acting this way?" he asks me.

"Dad is just trying to show you how to act normal," I answer.

"Quit defending him."

"She defends *you* all the time," says Jim. "Why can't she defend me?"

"As far as I can tell, I assume a needy..."

Jim: "Stance."

"Stance."

Jim: "Okay. I'll quit teasing. What did you think of dinner?"

"It was delicious."

"Dad used up some of the smell," complains Kevin, after his father had sniffed the wooden wick.

Jim: "Shall I light it and give it more smell?"

"Yes."

"I want to tease Dad because I love him," says Kevin, flicking the wick at his father.

"I tease *you* because I love you," says Jim.

"Is Dad angry at me?"

"No. Of course not."

As we leave the restaurant, Kevin stops to look at the live lobsters in the restaurant tank. "They can't be very happy," he types.

Later we ask our son, "What kind of day did you have today?"

"I'm glad we had such a special dinner."

"It was expensive," notes Jim.

"It was worth it. You can afford it. You have a good job. What time are we leaving?"

"Whenever we wake up," I say. "We'll visit Cornwallis and be at the ferry before noon."

## The continuum of our vulnerabilities

Kevin may occasionally mention his limitations, as when he spoke to his father about his "needy stance." But he doesn't usually dwell on this aspect of his life. Although he sometimes has to be reminded that all is well and that he needn't be anxious, he generally accepts who he is, and moves on to the next moment.

When Kevin was younger, I was overly concerned with the perceived stares and whispers of observers. Having my four little boys appear clean, nicely dressed and well behaved in public was very important to me. But life provides us with valuable lessons that can give direction whenever we are graced enough to recognize them. I received two such lessons when Kevin was ten. The first occurred while I was shopping for groceries with my youngest son, Joel.

Down one of the isles, a boy in a wheelchair was assisting a young woman with grocery shopping. The boy was about ten years old, and was obviously pleased with being included in the task.

For each item, the woman would hold the shopping list down to the boy's eye level and point to the desired word. The boy would scan the shelves carefully for the desired product, and then rise slowly on wobbly legs to reach it. Grasping the wheelchair arm tightly with his left hand, he would take the box or bottle from the shelf in his other hand and clutch it to his body. Painstakingly, he would then turn his torso to the left where the shopping cart was being steadied by the woman. Slowly, intently, he would extend his right arm over the cart and drop the grocery item.

"You're doing fine," the woman would comment quietly as the boy eased himself back into his chair. Or she would say, "That's great!" or some other words of warm encouragement.

Enchanted, I watched furtively from farther down the supermarket aisle.

"Look, Mommy. That boy has a chair with wheels," Joel announced with four-year-old naïveté. Naïveté, for even older children know that you do not stare at a handicapped person, much less call attention to his differences.

I took Joel's hand and we continued along, but the scene I had witnessed lingered in my mind. I was affected not by the disabled boy's appearance, but by the attitude of the woman who was shopping with him. She had seemed totally unconcerned about the glances of other customers. The boy and she were raptly occupied with the job of shopping and with each other. The attention she gave him was wholesome and happy, and he responded with unselfconscious enthusiasm. Moreover, their fellow shoppers were relaxed by the naturalness of their relationship. This was not a child to be pitied, or a mother with whom to commiserate.

My thoughts turned to my own disabled son. Straight of limb and with handsome features, his brain was imprisoned by the baffling condition known as autism. The third-born of our four sons, he had always been included in our family activities. Travelling, camping, zoos, museums, Sunday Masses – Kevin had enjoyed all these experiences with the rest of us.

But now a nagging doubt had stolen into my mind. I realized with some reluctance that I was not like the mother who accompanied the boy in the wheelchair. Whenever I felt the eyes of the public upon my autistic son, I became defensive and uncomfortable. I wanted them to see a well-behaved little boy, even though they seldom did. Instead they saw a boy who might suddenly snatch a piece of used gum from the sidewalk and pop it into his mouth.

They saw a child who would pick up string or a paper strip and, flicking it between his thumb and forefinger, would make it dance in snaky ripples. They saw a child who behaved unpredictably (to say the least) and an anxious mother who tried to hustle him along with as little fuss as possible.

Families of disabled persons feel that the community wishes to be spared the sight of a human being who does not fit their idea of normal. And we who have these challenged relatives are indeed guilty of going out of our way to make them less conspicuous.

But the experience in the supermarket prompted me to admit that I had ample room for improvement. I resolved to behave like the mother of the boy in the wheelchair when next I ventured into public view with Kevin.

Joel and I rounded a corner in the store, and there they were again, the boy and woman enjoying an outing. They were having such fun that their pleasure was infectious. Of course, the boy was not physically capable of leaping about and creating the type of mischief at which Kevin excelled. But even so, the cause-effect relationship was obvious. When a handicapped person is with someone who enjoys his company and, more importantly, shows it, onlookers are comfortable and have no reason to feel pity or embarrassment.

Joel and I wheeled our cart into the checkout line...and then I noticed them. Accompanied by adults who were undoubtedly their teachers, several children in braces and wheelchairs were lining up at the cash registers. It was obviously an educational outing for disabled children.

It wasn't his mother after all, I realized with keen disappointment. The young woman whom I had admiringly watched was carrying out a job, simply being professional.

But it doesn't have to be that way. It is harder for a mother to be objective about her own child, but it can be done.

The second lesson occurred a few days later. At the time, I was teaching piano, having changed careers from being an operating room nurse in order to accommodate my children's needs. It was early morning. Two of my young students had arrived to work on a duet. Kevin was still at home, awaiting the taxi that would take him to school.

"Hi, Kevin," they said, greeting him cautiously. Kevin ignored them, so the girls proceeded to organize their books at the piano. Now, an autistic child displays affection in much the same way as a cat does. Call a cat to sit on your lap, and it will trot demurely by as if you didn't exist. But try to read the paper or write a letter, and with a gentle push and persistent purr, there sits the feline between you and the paper, turning on affection and demanding attention.

And so it was with Kevin. No sooner had the music begun than he came and stood beside the young pianists. When they continued with the lesson, he patted one girl on the arm. This was too much, and she began to giggle. Embarrassed, she tried to hide the giggling behind her hand.

Usually, my music students caught only fleeting glimpses, if any, of Kevin, because at lesson time he was either at school or with a sitter-tutor. I wished the taxi would hurry and spare us all this discomfort.

But then the supermarket scene flashed through my mind. I remembered how we shoppers had been put at ease by the nonchalance of the handicapped boy and his companion. After all, they were merely engaging in a social function to which we are all entitled. By being themselves, they gave the rest of us the opportunity to accept them unconditionally. Did not the Creator intend that we should share the earth and its plenty? As social creatures, we are not fulfilled until we learn to give wholeheartedly and receive graciously.

Kevin wants to be accepted as he is, too, I thought. Through his distorted senses, he struggles to comprehend the bustling environment in which he dwells. Like the boy in the supermarket, he makes no apologies for his existence. Why, then, should I?

"Kevin must like your music," I volunteered.

"He must!" exclaimed the musicians, relieved to have the silence broken.

"You're funny, Kevin."

"You better be careful, Kevin, or you're going to get a lesson, too."

All uneasiness forgotten, the girls were laughing, and Kevin was joining in while jumping up and down in delight. The beeping of the taxi's horn interrupted the pleasant moment and, smiling happily, my son departed. The piano lesson continued, as did my enlightenment.

It might have been a day like any other. But it was not, for I had caught another sighting of a truth known by all children. Life is for sharing. Hurts do diminish when shared with sympathetic friends. Pleasure increases when divided among many.

This happy paradox had been acted out before my privileged eyes, first by a handicapped boy in the company of his guardian, and later by an autistic child and two young girls. As vibrant participants rather than aloof spectators, they demonstrated to me that fear and pride interfere with the natural flow of human acceptance. It would be another five years before I would become a Secular Franciscan. As a Franciscan, I would be called to examine more deeply fear and pride. I would be invited to dare to accept my human limitations. I would learn that "the ascent to God involves a descent into the obscure, dark regions within, so that the heights of the spirit coincide with the depths of the soul."[1]

But even though Jesus Christ took our humanity upon himself, we seem disinclined to accept human weakness. When Capuchin Professor William Hugo invites his students to say something negative about Francis of Assisi, he finds his students reluctant. He explains:

> If anything negative can be said, it usually is about the person before conversion, when limitations and sinfulness make for a more dramatic conversion to holiness. It's the "playboy to priest" syndrome. It makes for a great story.
>
> It's also an illusion. If we want to meet the historical Francis, we have to meet his limitations. If we don't, we will preoccupy ourselves with something that is not human and of doubtful help in our own lives. I never could identify with

the indestructible hero, the flawless leader, or the sinless saint. I'm none of those things and never will be.[2]

Another interesting feature of limitation is its position on the genetics spectrum. Temple Grandin says that people may angrily ask "why nature or God created such horrible conditions as autism, manic depression, and schizophrenia. However, if the genes that caused these conditions were eliminated there might be a terrible price to pay. It is possible that persons with bits of these traits are more creative, or possibly even geniuses."[3]

In addressing limitations, we might begin by examining our own. One of these might be the discomfort we feel around those living with illness, poverty, disabilities, addiction or homelessness. It is not always easy to see God in the lepers of society. Nor are we all disposed to become personally involved with marginalized people.

The hardest truth to learn could be that we are not suited for hands-on ministry with persons who are poor, homeless and vulnerable. Catherine Gugerty, who has worked in a homeless shelter and a soup kitchen, writes that "an even harder truth might be: I need to accept this truth and find a way in which I can still respond to the gospel mandate to be in solidarity with persons who are vulnerable." Gugerty goes on to say that if we lack the constitution for hands on involvement, we can instead "become advocates for those who have no voice in our society."[4]

Human limitation is repeatedly acknowledged in sacred Scripture. Some are slow and need help, lack strength and abound in poverty, notes the author of Sirach. But the eyes of the Lord look kindly upon them, "lifting them out of their lowly condition" (Sirach 11:12). From the end of the earth I call to you when "my heart is faint," cries the Psalmist. "Lead me to the rock that is higher than I, for you are my refuge, a tower against the enemy" (Psalm 61:2-3). The gospels contain many examples of Jesus' disciples being confounded by their weaknesses. In one such incident, we find them with Jesus in a boat, overtaken by a sudden storm. They wake him up, saying, "Lord, save us! *We are perishing!*" (Matthew 8:25).

St. Paul tells the Romans that he speaks to them in human terms because of their *natural limitations*. He tells us that we have peace with God through our Lord Jesus Christ. How can we not have peace when we are able to boast in our hope of sharing the glory of God? How can we not have peace when we can boast in our sufferings? "Now on first thought," says V.C. Keating, "I would rather have peace due to my hope of glory than in my sufferings. But Paul reminds us that suffering produces endurance which in turn produces character which then produces the hope of glory. And this hope does not disappoint us because God's wonderful love has been poured into our hearts through the Holy Spirit."[5]

Accepting limitations in ourselves and others is something we must tackle over and over. We are forever striving to rise above our human condition, but facing our humanity takes courage.

To be human is to be vulnerable and to have limitations. Jesus Christ honoured our humanity by taking it upon himself. We can help each other accept our frailties by reaching out with love and compassion. Within our families, we are challenged to recognize, accept and honour the strengths and weaknesses of each family member. At the same time, we cannot allow one child's limitations to overwhelm us with anxiety, or to consume all the family's time and energy.

Nor can we overlook the fact that dependency can be both cross and crutch. Along with the unavoidable dependency that persons with handicaps or chronic illness must endure, these same individuals are at high risk for developing dependent personalities. Such individuals

> surrender major decisions and responsibilities to others and permit the needs of those they depend on to supersede their own. They lack self-confidence and feel intensely insecure about their ability to take care of themselves. They often protest that they can't make decisions and don't know what to do or how to do it. They are reluctant to express opinions even when they have them for fear of offending people they need.[6]

It is the duty of parents to raise independent children. When our children have handicaps, this is more challenging. We often need divine intervention to encourage the highest attainable independence while at the same time teaching our children acceptance of their limitations. It is especially difficult to determine the capabilities of persons with autism.

Recently, I asked Kevin how he feels when he requires help with personal hygiene. He typed, "I feel a bit embarrassed and I hope the person doesn't mind, and I wish I could do it completely myself." Even here it is hard to determine how much of his difficulties stem from learned helplessness, dependent personality or the neurological havoc of autism.

"Do you think there is anything positive in it for the helper?" I asked. Solemnly, he replied, "Yes, if the person has a good attitude." Such an attitude grows out of genuine self-acceptance.

Once we have accepted our own limitations, says Sister Frances Teresa, "then we will not need to deny those of others, and so compassion comes alive in us. Our hearts open up to the world's pain in tender and redeemed solidarity, and we in our turn begin to show others clear footprints in which to place their feet."[7]

Kevin is a truly compassionate person, feeling deeply for people who suffer, as well as for all of God's creatures – including lobsters. On my best days I try to place *my* feet in *his* footprints, striving for solidarity with the world's pain.

**Spiritual journey**

Spiritual growth comes from viewing our limitations and our gifts as a small but vital part of the larger community of humankind. Our own joys, sufferings and vulnerability are part of humanity's joy, suffering and vulnerability. As Christians, we have the freedom to feel the pain that is part of being human, "the freedom to enter into solidarity with the suffering of the world precisely because [we are] sure of God's love."[8]

Francis of Assisi taught us that it's good to be small. It's okay to be a tiny particle in the vastness of creation. Vulnerable people do not expect to find fulfillment in material things, in power or in a career. They have to find this at a simpler, and therefore a deeper, level.

Persons with limitations have much to teach the world, and family members have front row seats. Kevin's brothers reflect on family life, and about their concerns over traits and genetics, now that they have children of their own.

> I guess the main reflections I have [says James] are that I'm thankful I have two healthy daughters, and that I still cannot fathom what Kevin and my parents went through (and continue to go through) on a daily basis. I now know that being a parent is difficult enough at the best of times.
>
> I would like to say that I wasn't concerned about genetics. However, as an educated individual who kept up on the scientific information on autism, I was. In fact, I did considerable research during university into the genetic characteristics of autism (which still remain elusive). Even though the odds were hugely in favour against having an autistic child, I held my breath during the first few years of my daughters' lives, looking for any indication of a problem. In fact, it wasn't until they had their fourth birthdays that I convinced myself we were in the clear.
>
> The risk of developmental disabilities was a factor in Laurie and I not having a third child, albeit only one of many factors. I do think that Kevin being the third child spooked us a bit, even though there is no logic behind it.
>
> Now that I have my own children [notes Chris], I have come to understand the power that they hold over you. I can understand how motivated parents can be when trying to provide the best possible life for their child regardless of whether that child has a developmental disability. I have had concerns about traits and genetics. Both my spouse and I have a sibling with a developmental disability. When Jodi was pregnant with our first child, I was worried. I knew my fears were not rational, as I understood that our siblings' types of disabilities were not related to genetics, and there

was little increased risk of having a child with disabilities.[9] Everything turned out fine.

Six years later, Jodi became pregnant with our second child. Throughout this second pregnancy I had a bad, nagging feeling, which of course was irrational, that we had dodged a bullet the first time and that we shouldn't have tempted fate again. Our second child is now eleven months old and, so far, everything is fine. I suppose these are concerns that all parents experience. I don't know if I shared the same fears of every expectant parent or if my fears were heightened because of my family history.

Joel has had an even more harrowing experience. After his wife, Heather, had suspicious blood test and ultrasound results, she and Joel were sent for genetic counselling. They were told that there was a high likelihood of their unborn child having spina bifida or a chromosomal abnormality. Spina bifida is a spinal cord defect in which part of one or more vertebrae fails to develop completely, leaving a portion of the spinal cord unprotected. Effects of this condition range from none to total paralysis, depending on how severely the spinal cord and nerve roots are affected. Although they were greatly concerned, Joel and Heather would not consider abortion, and therefore refused the recommended amniocentesis used to further detect abnormalities in a fetus. All of this was very upsetting for them. As Joel explains,

> Our son, Aidan, had a rough start to his life – spending seven weeks in neonatal intensive care units. He has had genetic screening, so genetics is naturally a concern to me. However, I was never really that concerned about autism during my wife's pregnancy, with all the other possibilities being suggested, such as spina bifida. Generally though, having Kevin as a brother hasn't really changed how I would live my family life, or the choices I would make.

Aidan still has some health issues, but he is a bright, happy little boy with no spina bifida or chromosomal abnormalities.

"Because there is some evidence of a genetic factor in autism," adds Jim, "I have been concerned that our boys and their spouses would be worried at every pregnancy. I was also concerned about Gloria's sisters and parents, because I knew they would worry over every family pregnancy. They were so involved with Kevin. Everyone has seemed to handle it well, at least as far as I know."

Hoping for a healthy baby, and fearing that something may go wrong, are experiences of every parent. Life is riddled with uncertainties. Rohr reminds us that instead of certainties, Jesus gives us a faith journey. Instead of answers, he tells us what the right questions are. By not having all the answers, we are dependent on each other. "The real meaning of a poor life is a life of radical dependency."[10]

To acknowledge dependency is to be poor in spirit. "Blessed are the poor in spirit," Jesus says (Matthew 5:3). In surrendering to our need for God and each other, we acquire the peace and joy of Francis and Clare. We ally our darkness, fears and limitations with the humanity of Christ, and nestle into the heart of God. Thus we free ourselves from needless worry, adopting a sense of trust and acceptance that all is well and all will be well.

As our lives unfold, we take into our beings the anguish and joy that we encounter in ourselves and others. These experiences influence and change the way we view things. William Hugo describes how Francis' changing vision of life outside himself began to change his vision of life within himself. Francis began to ask the common human question, 'Why me?' But he asked this question from an unusual perspective. "Generally, this query in life asks why pain and suffering happen to me, as if somehow I am unjustly sentenced to singular or disproportionate struggle," Hugo says. Francis, on the other hand, "asked why he was not suffering in light of all the suffering around him."[11]

To view our suffering as small within the sea of suffering around us, to see our limitations as less than those of others, to accept our gifts and talents as few among many: this is spiritual growth.

# 9

# Pioneers and Pilgrims

**From Kevin's journal: Day 17**

Day 17 – August 2, 1992 – Digby and St. John

"I'm happy we're going on the ferry," announces Kevin this morning. "When are we leaving?"

"As soon as we can go aboard," I say. "Where is your smoke stick?"

"I forgot about it. Can I keep it?"

"Do you think it will help you avoid butts?"

"I think it's worth a try."

When we reach the location of the Digby ferry, I ask him, "Do you want to get out?"

"Yes. Where are we going?"

"Inside the terminal."

"I will stay here, then."

"We're going to be here for quite a while."

"OK. I'll go with Dad for a bit."

Kevin and his father wander around for a while before returning to the car. We are then approached by the ferry surveyor who asks, "Does anyone collect pins? Kevin does? Well, here's a city pin for you."

"Thank you very much," types Kevin. "That's very kind of you."

Impressed by Kevin's ability, the ferry surveyor adds, "I have another special pin just for you," and hands him a different pin of Digby.

"That's great."

Sitting in the car a while longer, we ask Kevin, "Do you prefer the stick or the tobacco?"

"I think the stick is much better."

Jim suggests that he and Kevin go to the washroom. They soon return in a state of thinly suppressed agitation. Jim is furious because Kevin had broken away from him in order to dash ahead to eat a butt.

"Why did you behave so badly for Dad?" I ask Kevin.

"I didn't have to go to the washroom, and I didn't like walking in front of all those people. It was too frightening."

"Why did you run away and eat a butt?"

"That's what I do when I'm upset." Kevin always has an excuse.

"Well, what about Dad? He's upset, too."

"I'm sorry I upset him. As far as I can tell, I should try to act better."

"You certainly should. Dad looks about ready to cry."

"Tell him I'm sorry. I didn't mean to embarrass him."

We manage to calm down sufficiently to settle into our cabin. We are determined to not let addiction ruin our vacation.

"Do you like our cabin?" I ask.

"It's very nice. I think I will want to go on the deck sometime."

"And how will you behave?"

"As far as I can tell, I will behave well."

"I'm going now," says Jim. "Do you want to come?"

"Leave me here, please. Then perhaps I will go out when the ferry moves. This is boring."

"We'll be here for two-and-a-half hours. Do you want to go with Dad?"

"Yes."

Kevin and Jim enjoy an uneventful stroll through the ferry. When they return, we have a snack, but Kevin does not want to eat. "Captain asked us not to eat in our cabin," he says by way of explanation.

"No. It's all right," says Jim. "We can eat here."

"As far as I can tell, people are to eat in the cafeteria."

"I think the captain said we can't eat in our *cars*," I say.

"As far as I can tell, we're breaking rules. We better not eat."

"The captain said cars, not cabins," insists Jim. "It's fine to eat here."

"Are you enjoying the ferry?" I ask.

"It's perhaps making me sick."

"Come and lie down then."

"As far as I can tell, I'm better sitting upright."

"The ferry to Newfoundland is much longer. One way is six hours, and the other one is twelve hours."

"That would be great." Kevin knows that we had been unable to book passage to Newfoundland prior to the trip as we had wished.

"What if you get sick?" I ask.

"Then I would lie down and sleep."

After we disembark at St. John, New Brunswick, we ask Kevin, "Did you enjoy the ferry?"

"Yes," he replies. "It was good except for the rolling which made me a bit sick."

Sometime later, we stop to eat. Kevin is in a playful mood. "What do you want?" I ask.

"I want to bug you."

"That's what I thought."

When I question Kevin about his obsessive nose stimming, he first replies, "I pick my nose because it feels stuffy."

But when I persist, he says, "Never mind about my nose. Perhaps it is *my* nose. I will try to use Kleenex."

"Dad wants to know if you know what he does for a living."

"He is of course a principal."

"Where?"

"Of St. Philip's School. Why did Dad think I wouldn't know that?"

"Is principal a good job?" persists Jim.

"You should know the answer to that," said Kevin.

"But I want to hear *your* answer," says his father.

"As far as I can tell, it pays very well and has great benefits."

"What puzzles me," remarks Jim, "is how you can be so smart and behave as badly as you did this morning."

"You have to understand that's one of the unfortunate symptoms of autism. I don't do well in crowds."

"Yes, I understand that," says Jim. "What kind of restaurant is this?"

"As far as I can tell, it's a strange restaurant."

"It's Mexican," explains Jim.

"Yes," agrees Kevin. "I didn't understand the question."

"Do you want to walk downtown St. John?" I ask.

"That will be fun."

"The crowds won't bother you?"

"It will probably be fine because the people will be watching the entertainment and not me."

"How do you know there's entertainment?" asks Jim.

"I saw the crowd and heard you talking about the clowns."

"Did we tell your mother about the boy on the ferry who asked all the questions about you?" asks Jim.

"I dare say he was greatly curious about me. I was embarrassed by being made to perform signs for him. As far as I can tell, I have some dignity and should be able to ignore kids."

"Dad was only letting the boy know how smart you are," I suggest.

"Dad meant well but he shouldn't have involved me. Dad likes to entertain but I don't."

After dinner, we go walking. "Look at the busker with his music machine!" I exclaim.

"This is incredible," types Kevin. "He has everything going at once."

"Did you see what the monkey did?" I ask.

"It peed."

"What do you think of this?" asks Jim.

"It's quite unique. We are lucky to have happened by when this is taking place."

"For sure," I agree.

On our way back to our room, Jim asks Kevin, "Did you remember seeing the Martello Tower?"

"We saw it on our way to the Reversing Falls. There was not much to see."

"Do you remember the magnetic hill?" asks Jim.

"Yes. That was when we were in New Brunswick earlier. It was better than the Reversing Falls."

"Do you remember being in the Special Olympics?" I now ask Kevin, wanting an explanation for some things that had happened in his past.

"Yes," he replies.

The first Special Olympics competitions, although held in Chicago in 1968, were the results of the efforts of Dr. Frank Hayden, a Toronto researcher and professor. Dr. Hayden's efforts to develop a national Canadian sports program for intellectually disabled people caught the attention of Eunice Kennedy Shriver and the

Kennedy Foundation in Washington, D.C. Testing of children with developmental disabilities in the '60s indicated that they were only half as physically fit as their non-disabled peers. Challenging this assumption, Hayden developed an intense fitness program and "demonstrated that, given the opportunity, intellectually disabled people could become physically fit and acquire the physical skills necessary to participate in sport. His research proved that low levels of fitness and lack of motor skills development in people with mental handicaps were a result of nothing more than a sedentary lifestyle."[1]

"Do you know why you didn't try to win when you were such an excellent runner?" I ask.

"I didn't understand that I was supposed to win by myself."

"But we would all scream and yell at you to run!"

"I'm sorry I disappointed you."

"It was your peer tutor that I felt sorry for. He worked so hard with you."

"Yes. I let him down."

"Why did you not run fast?"

"I thought I was just supposed to race for fun."

"Will you be in the Special Olympics again?"

"I hope so. I will win for sure because I am faster than most people."

"Why didn't you run fast before?"

"They didn't explain it right. They told me I should have fun and not worry about winning. They didn't want to have me worrying and getting upset. But they were too kind and I let them down."

"There was kindness on your part also, Kevin. In Windsor, I saw you deliberately wait for the last racer so you could run in with her."

"Yes. I didn't want to leave her by herself."

"Did you know her?"

"As far as I can tell, I didn't know her, but I still felt sorry for her."

"How many Olympics were you in?"

"Four, I think."

"And you won some medals," I reassure him.

"Yes. I sometimes won, but I could have done much better. I am a sad person."

"Don't be a sad person. That's past, and it's never a loss when we learn from experience. You didn't understand the concept of competition."

"Besides," adds Jim, "you were kind and that is most important."

"I'm happy I understand now. I'm glad that you and Dad, as far as I can tell, are not disappointed in me, and that you don't think I'm a loser."

"We're very proud of you."

"When am I going back to St. Francis House?"

"Next Saturday."

"As far as I can tell, that's good. I've had a wonderful holiday with you, and I'm looking forward to school. Thank you for explaining that to me. Will I go on holidays with you and Dad next summer?"

"Certainly."

"That's great. Where will we go?"

"We haven't planned that far ahead."

"What about Newfoundland?"

"We'll either go next year or the following summer."

"That's great."

## Parents as pioneers and pilgrims

Sometimes it seems that, as parents, we go from crisis to crisis. Having a child with autism has certainly taken us through valleys that were indeed shadowed. Take something as simple as swimming lessons.

Before Kevin's illness became apparent, we had enrolled him in an infant swim course. Somehow his swimming ability survived the onset of autism, and swimming gave him tremendous pleasure. Kevin's love of water, however, soon became a frequent source of chagrin.

In search of water, Kevin wandered from campsites, shopping malls, and the homes of alarmed friends and relatives. Throughout Canada and the United States, he set off widespread search parties consisting of friends and strangers alike. As well, he often managed to slip away from our home to go swimming in private pools near and far.

It was not at all unusual, in spite of my constant vigilance, for me to get a phone call telling me to come and claim my dripping son. Dropping everything, I would dash frantically to the designated address. If it were too far away, I would have to call Jim home from his school.

On some occasions, sympathetic people would be comforting the poor lost boy with cookies. More often, I would be berated by irate pool owners who'd been thoroughly frightened by the discovery of a small boy splashing (and presumed drowning) in a pool surrounded by a six-foot fence with a padlocked gate.

From an early age, Kevin had remarkable climbing skills. As well as scaling pool enclosures, he had no hesitation in climbing *any* fence. On one occasion, a neighbour banged frantically on my door and told me to come at once. Three houses up the street lived a young couple who had in their backyard a fenced run for their German shepherds. These dogs would let no one near when the owners were not home. One of the dogs was especially agitated at this time because, while the owners worked, she was separated from her new litter of pups, which were safely indoors.

There, playing at the feet of these dogs, was Kevin! Even worse, the dogs were protecting Kevin from *us* with hysterical barking and vicious snarling. A gathering of horrified neighbours helplessly watched as I tried to coax Kevin out. Eventually, Kevin was enticed by a cookie, and nonchalantly clambered over the fence, oblivious to the alarm he had created. It was just another day in the life of a little boy with autism (and of his perplexed mother).

When one member of the family is more limited than the others, or any member is ill, it's natural to focus on that person. This is fine for a short-term situation, but for a chronic condition, such individualized attention becomes unhealthy for everyone.

Some of the parents we encountered in similar situations over the years withdrew into their misery. Despairing, distrusting and resentful, they seemed unable to seek help, participate in parent support groups, or lobby for better conditions for themselves and their children. They wrapped their lives around their vulnerable child and hunkered fearfully in the valley that was their lot.

Others threw themselves into the whirlwind of modern life. They involved their children in various lessons: piano, violin, swimming, soccer, skating. They sought out the latest therapies: megavitamin, allergy, diet, patterning. They attended meetings and conferences near and far. They lobbied and laboured. They rushed and ran. The vulnerable child was swept along in the activities of his siblings in the hope that he would become like them.

Our family fit mostly into the latter category. Would I do things differently today? Probably not a whole lot – just because I'm me. But I would definitely try to keep our lives simpler and I would consult my children more on their own choices. I would allow more for individuality, encouraging each child to nurture his or her own talents. I would recognize that children, as well as parents, can become overextended and worn out.

I would acknowledge that living simply involves rejecting materialism in its many guises within possessions and lifestyle. As pilgrims on the journey of life, we should possess as little as possible, and regularly assess our needs.

## Spiritual journey

Although we have little control over many of the happenings in our lives, these events contribute to our makeup. How we integrate these experiences determines who we become.

The Psalmist tells us that, rather than seeing ourselves as moving from crisis to crisis, we are to go "from strength to strength." As our pilgrimage takes us through the fearful "valley of Baca," we are to make it a "place of springs." The confidence we have in our difficult journey comes from our God of mercy and strength. As we tread the "highways to Zion," we know that God travels with us (Psalm 84:6-7).

We make our family journey a place of springs by recognizing our strengths and weaknesses. We acknowledge our weaknesses, but build on our strengths and go from strength to strength. The family unit itself is the greatest strength. As well as being the basic building block of society, it is the source of nurturing, mentoring and protection. It's the means of celebrating accomplishments and solving problems.

"Kevin gave me insight into life that only families of a disabled and/or addicted person can gain," says James. "I now understand that being in a loving environment, working hard, being dedicated and pursuing knowledge sometimes isn't enough to avoid significant pitfalls in life. Anyone can become disabled anytime. Anyone can become addicted to something anytime. Take what life gives you in stride as best you can, and with support from those around you and God willing, you will get through it."

"In many ways I am a stronger and better person having grown up with Kevin," agrees Chris. "I believe that I am more understanding and tolerant of people with disabilities than the average person is out there.

"This is not to say that some of Kevin's behaviours, particularly those associated with addictions (such as slipping over to the neighbour's place to sniff gas) weren't a source of embarrassment to me, from time to time."

"Yes," adds Joel. "I remember waking up, or being awakened, as a child so we could go on a manhunt to find out where Kevin had stolen off to in the middle of the night. This certainly made sleeping peacefully at night a little more difficult."

"I used to think I was hard done by," observes Chris. "As I've grown older, I'm not sure these difficulties were any harder to bear than difficulties faced by many other families who are confronted with problems in their families such as divorce, alcoholism, drug addiction, poverty, or mental illness."

My adult children accept that the events of their childhoods have contributed to their strength and goodness. Experiences happy and sad, pleasant and difficult, have made them who they are. Throughout their lives they will continue to acquire confidence, wisdom, expertise and new insights. They will recognize themselves as pioneers, using their God-given creativity and talents to blaze new paths for the enrichment of others. They will see themselves as pilgrims, travelling in protective, encouraging bands across the lands and seas of life.

Living courageously as pioneers and travelling lightly as pilgrims requires practice, patience and grace. Andrew Bloomfield, a young man with autism, observes, "I like being a pioneer but it is too slow and scary sometimes."[2] Beginnings tend to be slow and scary, and in new situations, caution is the prudent course of action.

Speaking about the beginnings of L'Arche in 1964, Jean Vanier says that his role "was to welcome events as they came and let them guide me. Later I discovered that my ignorance and poverty at the beginning of L'Arche helped me be more attentive to God, and let him guide me from day to day. Had I had a clear plan, I might have been less ready to welcome God's plan."[3]

Insecurity allows us to be more genuinely open to God's action. When everything seems to fall smoothly into place, we begin to think we have less need for God. "Life becomes comfortable, and enthusiasm wanes," says Vanier. "Those who get in the way are excluded. People are less present to others; they think more about themselves."[4]

There are indeed challenges in taking on the role of either pioneer or pilgrim. Searching far and wide for answers, we are willing to risk danger and ridicule. Constantly seeking a better life, "a better place, a greater state of wellbeing, we are always somewhat restless and vaguely discontent," notes V.C. Keating.[5] We grow to accept, as St. Augustine did, that only in God will we find total peace, and only in heaven will we be completely at rest.

In doing so, we model hope. By our efforts we demonstrate that everyone can live life on earth to the fullest as an integral part of our pilgrimage home to God. We demonstrate that there can be satisfaction, even joy, in the journey. As pioneers and pilgrims, our lives are inspired by all people of faith who have gone before us. Through pleasant wanderings and unavoidable trials, we are cheered on by witnesses seen and unseen. Keeping our sights on Jesus, who endured hostility and humiliation for us, we have the strength to persevere. Because the way has been prepared for us, it is our duty to pass along peace, encouragement and holiness to those who journey with us and after us.

If in this world we are already living in the reign of God, writes Rohr, "then the world becomes relative and we become 'pilgrims and strangers.' Life can't be based on transitory images. Instead we know we have to base it on the truth, on the truth of who we are, on the truth of this creation, which God says is 'very good.'"[6]

Yes, God is good, and those of us who are blessed with the companionship of the poor in spirit have a wonderful opportunity to illuminate this blessing to the world. We have the means of showing our discovery – their beauty and wisdom – to a troubled world.

St. Clare teaches us that social discernment includes listening to the minority voice, because God often reveals what is best to the one who is the least. Sister Frances Teresa explains,

> God is still at work in our technological world, still creating it from within, still giving it possibilities and a future. As always, we are invited to bring the Gospel into that world, sharing our best with it as God shared the Word with us. We have a task of discernment and Clare teaches us how to do it. Guided by her, we learn to discern the Spirit of the Lord and his holy manner of working, and against this work, we assess our own.[7]

To live Franciscan spirituality is to pursue simplicity, the poverty of Francis and Clare. "The more things you need, the less free you are," writes Adela Torchia. "Asceticism is not masochism! Asceticism means saying no to all the things that claim to be crucial for your happiness but which in fact are a burden and a distraction."[8]

Along with placing our material possessions in proper perspective, we must also evaluate our use of time. This is my greatest struggle. I want to be everything and do everything, which may explain, at least partly, the variety in my past careers. Much of this has been a blessing, but it has also been a source of restlessness and, sometimes, anxiety. Lately I remind myself frequently that God is not asking me to fill each day with non-stop activity, but only to trustingly place myself in God's hands.

Among Christians, there are those who act and those who pray. We are best suited for one or the other, but we work away on our shadow selves in order to find a balance between the two – to be more Christ-like. Those of us who are driven to be doers seem to be always struggling with our prayer lives.

It's true that Secular Franciscans are called to live in the world and not on their knees in a remote chapel. But it's also true that we are called to be people of prayer, to live the gospel. We can only really do that when we detach ourselves from all that distracts us from the reality of our journey. As pioneers and pilgrims, we travel a continuum that stretches from time to eternity.

Our earth journey as we know it has its difficulties and then it will end. Patti Normile writes that "excessive pleasure-seeking, consumerism, abuse of alcohol, drugs or food are all human attempts to dodge life's realities. When we understand that this lifetime is but a speck on the eternal time line, we begin to attend to the real business of living the gospel."[9]

Thérèse of Lisieux meditated on the biblical texts in which God proclaims his preferential love for those who have the heart of a child. She then developed a style of praying, "The Little Way," which described

> a path that everyone can follow, a life without ecstasies or special penances.... Thérèse understood early that to attain sanctity, it is not necessary to do outstanding works.... She especially understood that, to unite oneself to God in truth, one must first of all let oneself be found, loved and fashioned by him. His love is the gratuitous love of a father for his children. He always loves us first.[10]

As prayer leads to union with God, so prayer

intrinsically and invariably leads to union with all people and all creation. That is why the work of prayer and the work of justice are so essentially related. One cannot truly know God and self in the silence of personal prayer without also knowing God and self in the suffering, anguish and despair of humanity and our violated earth. The only appropriate response to such knowing is involvement.[11]

Prayer calls us to those who need us most; it leads us to those whom we most need.

And so we come full circle. Our relationship with God and our compassion for the earth and its people are inseparable. This is why we cannot be other than pioneers and pilgrims. As pioneers, we are compelled to lead. As pilgrims, we are committed to follow. All people – regardless of ability or disability, race, culture or creed – hear the same call and have the same needs. In respecting each other's differences, we welcome all fellow travellers as equals.

# 10

# The Quest for Meaning

**From Kevin's journal: Days 18 to 20**

*Day 18 – August 3, 1992 – St. John*

"What are we doing today?" Kevin wonders.

"We're spending another day here," I say.

"That sounds good. We need a day of rest."

"Dad deserves a rest. He's done all the driving and he planned the trip beforehand."

"Dad has done an excellent job of planning this trip. He deserves a rest," agrees Kevin.

At lunch, Jim comments on the restaurant. "This is an expensive place."

"I noticed that," says Kevin, adding, "and remember I have contributed to this trip."

"It's good you're helping out, Kevin," agrees his dad.

"Are you still mad?" Kevin asks me.

"I have to admit that I am," I say. "You just ate another butt and I reminded you not to like you asked me to."

"As far as I can tell, you have a right to be angry."

"What are we to do with you?"

"As far as I can tell, I am a sad person. Are you going to help me?"

"We are trying to help."

"Don't give up."

"You have to help yourself."

"I will try to help. As far as I can tell, I'm glad that I have improved."

"And you must continue to improve."

"Yes, I will continue to improve."

When we visit another museum, I ask Kevin, "What do you prefer here?"

"Perhaps the art. It's quite interesting, don't you think?"

As the day continues, I inquire of Kevin, "How many butts have you had so far today?"

"Four."

"Is there an explanation?"

"As far as I can tell, it's because I was upset."

"You made a face as you ate it. It must have tasted awful."

"It was good tasting."

"There are addicts living on the street. They collect butts, too. Did you know that?"

"No, I didn't."

"They eat garbage and sleep on newspapers because they can't keep family or friends or a job. Do you want to end up like that?"

"That would be terrible. Who would look after me?"

"No one."

"As far as I can tell, I would get sick."

Jim: "Yes. All addicts are sick."

"There are shelters that take in as many as possible on cold winter nights," I inform Kevin.

"That's good. Then they could have a meal and shower."

"Would you like to be a street person?"

"As far as I can tell, I would be unhappy. I will shape up."

"Where is your smoke stick?"

"I forgot it. It would have helped."

We then tour the New Brunswick Museum, where Kevin soon states, "I'm bored."

"This is a wonderful place full of fascinating tidbits from the past," I tell him. "Come and read this. What are these Tingqi bowls and pans for?"

"So the spirits would have things for their use."

"And the horse?"

"They could ride the horse."

"Does our religion believe this?"

"No. We believe that God will provide for us," says Kevin.

"Read what it says about the lion head on the horse."

"It was protection against evil spirits and thieves."

"Oh, look! There are more of these," I note.

"Yes, figureheads for ships."

"Did you hear the guide say these fossils were snail tracings?" I ask.

"I never would have guessed that," says Kevin. "I thought fossils were animals. Why is the black bear brown?"

"Let's ask the guide," says Jim.

Guide: "It has faded with age. But they're not really black anyway."

"Where have you seen furniture like this before?" I ask Kevin.

"At Louisbourg."

As we walk down the street sometime later, we pass a raggedy man, shuffling along with bowed head. "Look, there's a street person," I say to Kevin. "He's probably looking for butts just like you."

"That's not funny. I'm not like them. I'm cultured and come from a good family."

"Many of them have come from good families, too. But they've become addicts, and this is how they end up."

"That's terrible. I will not continue with my addiction. I don't know why I ate four butts today. I will take my smoke stick tomorrow and see if that helps."

"Kevin, did you just eat another butt?!" I am exasperated.

"Yes."

"I can't believe it! You *must* want to become a derelict."

"I would never want to do that. Why doesn't someone help them?"

"From time to time they commit a crime, and then they're put in prison or a psychiatric hospital. But soon they're back out on the streets."

"That's terrible. Do they have families?"

"Their families have lost touch with them."

"As far as I can tell, it's lucky I have a family. Are you and Dad angry?"

"Dad is very upset."

"Yes, I think he's really fed up," agrees Kevin.

Jim: "I'm not so much angry as sad."

"I'm sorry I upset Dad. Also I'm frightened I'm poisoning my body. Will you and Dad still help me?"

"Of course. Do you feel that you are getting more able to control yourself?"

"Yes, I think that I'm getting more confident that I can stop soon. Tomorrow will be a butt-free day."

That evening I say, "You seem to be getting more snugly, Kevin. Do you think you are?"

"Up until now I couldn't stand being hugged and kissed. But suddenly I like perhaps some hugging and kissing."

"Why might this be?"

"As far as I can tell, it must be because I'm more normal. My skin is not as sensitive."

People with autism receive skewed sensory messages from their brains. They can be hypersensitive or hyposensitive to touch, sound, light, taste or smell. They may shrink from bright light, loud sounds or certain textures. They may spit out food that has a certain taste or feel upon their tongues. On the other hand, they may crave a food with strong taste and smell, such as onions. They may be drawn to the sound of a vacuum cleaner or love the sight of swirling water in a toilet bowl. They may hate the feel of certain clothes against their skin or be so in need of sensory stimulation that they will deliberately touch a hot stove element.

Most likely, their senses will be a mixture of hyper and hypo. As a child, Kevin seemed to be acutely sensitive to loud sounds and bright light, while lacking in the sensory areas of taste, smell and touch. Thus he would ingest anything that caught his attention even if it were something vile. He also seemed immune to physical pain, gulping down scalding coffee, and not crying or even wincing over skinned knees.

As they mature, people with autism tend to adapt to their sensory extremes, but some abnormalities always seem to remain. Contrary to popular opinion, they can be very compassionate, empathetic and affectionate. However, they seldom manifest any of these emotions through their body language. Snugly they are not. But Kevin will tolerate *some* hugs and kisses at family gatherings. Sometimes he will even smile indulgently and return a stiff, arm's-length hug. He would prefer to shake hands.

*Day 19 – August 4, 1992 – Bangor, Maine*

"Why did you have such a bad night?" I ask the next day.

"I'm upset that Dad is mad at me."

"And you know why he was angry."

"Yes, but I was out of control."

"Why do you suppose you got out of control?"

"I was bored."

"Well, today is another day. You can make a fresh start."

"OK. I will try. Where are we going?"

"We'll be driving through Maine. It should be scenic and relaxing."

"Good. Am I going with you on your next summer holidays?"

"That will depend entirely on you. We will not tolerate another summer of butts." Undoubtedly, we are the classic enablers: always threatening, and then relenting.

"I will definitely get it under control. Are you mad at me?"

"No."

"Good, because I am a sad person."

"Sometimes one has to be a sad person in order to become a wiser person."

"I am wiser. I want you and Dad to love me."

"We will always love you."

"The TV is saying that people don't want developmentally handicapped people living in their neighbourhoods," notices Kevin suddenly. "They are narrow-minded people."

"They are ignorant and don't know any better," I say. "Perhaps you will help educate them."

"As far as I can tell, that's needed," agrees Kevin. "My writing will give them understanding."

"Are you okay now?"

"Yes, I'm happier."

"We should have a pleasant day."

"Yes, it should be perhaps great. I will certainly not do butts today," promises Kevin.

"What are we waiting for?" asks Kevin later while his father is inside a store. "Perhaps I should go in. I'm bored."

"Dad's looking for film and a New Brunswick pin for you."

"Okay. When are we leaving Canada? Great. I'm looking forward to Maine. I am happy. I love you."

But as we drive on, Kevin types, "You told me this would be a beautiful drive and it's ugly."

"We can't help it if it's foggy and rainy."

"Perhaps I should have a real New Brunswick pin."

"We will keep looking. What did you think of Father Rohr's tape?" I ask. We had been listening to an audiotape in the car.

"Not perhaps helpful."

"Why?"

"He should have told us to stop our addictions. He said it was not our fault."

"He said blaming oneself does no good."

"But whose fault is it?"

"It's the fault of original sin and our weak, sinful nature. Father Rohr said the important factor is naming our addiction and admitting we have it."

"What happens when you admit it?"

"You admit your helplessness and surrender to Jesus."

"And let Jesus help you."

"Right. Are you enjoying Maine more?"

"Yes, it's pleasant."

*Day 20 – August 5, 1992 – Rumford, New Hampshire*

"I'm feeling great," says Kevin. "Where are we going?"

"We'll still be travelling in Maine."

"Will we be staying at this motel?"

"No, we'll be further on. First, though, we'll be doing some shopping in Bangor."

Later, Kevin, knowing the answer, asks, "Will I be having coffee for lunch?"

"No. You just ate a butt."

"That's fair."

And later, more of the same. When Jim and Kevin exit a washroom at the Bangor Mall, Jim says, "He ate a butt out of the urinal."

"Kevin, I am disgusted!" I say.

"I can understand it. I know it's terrible. Do I get coffee for supper?"

"No."

"I'm sorry today has been a three-butt day. I will have to forget about coffee. You will have to watch me better. I can't seem to control myself. I hope my counsellor can come up with something."

In our motel room that night, Kevin types, "I'm angry that you reminded me that we have only three more nights."

"Would you rather be surprised?"

"As far as I can tell, I already know."

"How did you like the soup?" I ask out of curiosity, referring to our supper.

"It was fine but it tasted like condensed milk."

"I agree. When have you tasted condensed milk?"

"At home in coffee sometimes."

"I want my *People* magazine," says Jim to Kevin, who then hands it to his father. "When you riffled through it just now," asks Jim, "did you read anything?"

"There was an article on the Olympics people."

"Was there?" I ask.

"I don't know," says Jim. "I haven't found it yet. Yes, there it is!" Kevin continues to surprise us with his abilities. This undoubtedly prods our determination to help him overcome his addictions.

## Vocational hunger

"O God, I seek you, my soul thirsts for you; my flesh faints for you as in a dry and weary land" (Psalm 63:1). This longing, expressed so eloquently by the Psalmist some five centuries before the birth of Jesus, exists at the core of our beings. Planted within us at the beginning of our earthly lives, it persistently draws us towards the Creator.

Throughout our lives we feel the steady, patient pull of God in many ways. God's magnetism is in our desire for goodness, love, companionship and justice. It abides in our yearning for wisdom, knowledge and truth. We experience it in our curiosity about far-off places and distant planets. It beats within the stirring of our hearts at the sight of a peaceful lake at sunset or the sound of the haunting cry of a loon.

The beauty and workings of creation demand human interaction. We are not designed to be content watching the world pass us by. The Creator expects us to leave an imprint as we make our way along the paths of life. As we walk towards God and with God, we gain knowledge as we accumulate experience.

Every experience enriches our life in some way. One day, when I was writing in the peacefulness of a provincial park, I contemplated how pleasant a park ranger's life would be. My paternal grandfather, who died a couple of months before I was born, had been a park warden for a time. Too bad I hadn't followed his example, I thought. Then it occurred to me that my knowledge would be about flora and fauna, rather than health care, social services and parish dynamics. Perhaps I would still be writing today, but the subject matter would be entirely different.

Every person has the possibility of several careers and lifestyles. Some of us have more opportunities for choice. This can be because of the twists and turns in the road of our journey. Or it can be due to the abilities and disabilities with which we are equipped.

It remains a continuing challenge for Kevin and for us who assist him to keep his lifestyle meaningful. We try to have variety in his life, a mix of work and leisure, socializing and privacy, pleasant living with his two housemates, and regular family visiting. Because Kevin enjoys being with us so much, we welcome him for extended overnight stays and include him in our holidays and travelling.

We all enjoy learning and experiencing new things throughout our lives. Kevin is no exception. After all, do not the scriptures tell us that "the sincere desire for instruction is the beginning of wisdom" (Wisdom 6:17)? To attain wisdom is to grow ever closer to the love-saturated perfection of God. Thus all persons have the right to ongoing education.

In the fall of 1992, following the trip described in Kevin's journal, Kevin was trying to settle into his school routine, and we were attempting to wean him from needing a facilitator for typing. We hoped that wearing something around his wrist would provide a sensation similar to the touch of a person, thereby encouraging independent typing.

"Why am I wearing this wristband?" asked Kevin suspiciously.

"It's not a wristband. It's a wrist support," I said.

"As far as I can tell, it's strange," said Kevin. Later he added, "As far as I can tell, it's a silly-looking thing and the students will laugh."

"It's a medical support."

"It's a medical support and they will think I'm sick," he retorted.

"They'll think you have a muscular weakness. Would you rather they think you're not smart?" I said.

"I would rather they think I was a normal, intelligent person."

"I wish you had seen the TV documentary about the surgeon with Tourette's Syndrome," I told him. "He had all sorts of bizarre behaviours, but people still knew he was an intelligent doctor. It's the same with autism. They will get to understand that you are intelligent but have some difficulties."

"But it's weird," said Kevin, referring again to the wrist support.

"It's really not weird. Your dad and I searched all over Toronto for this support because we're sure it will help."

"I'm glad you got it for me."

"It's going to take practice but you can do it," I said.

"Yes. I'm glad you explained it to me. As far as I can tell, it will work fine. I will try hard."

"And you will win! You're a fighter and you can do it."

"Yes. I will try hard until I become an expert."

Despite occasional outbursts of frustration, Kevin is admirably courageous and determined. In the distorted world of autism, his life is full of trials and challenges from morning till night. Kevin is only too aware of his limitations and the resultant need for assistance from others in many areas of his life.

Unlike most students, he requested homework so that he would have time to complete it properly. "I cannot write quickly," he said, "but I have an excellent memory."

Yes, Kevin does have an excellent memory, and several other gifts. As well as having courage, determination and a fine memory, he is caring, compassionate and loyal. He has a keen sense of social justice for the poor, homeless, disabled and handicapped. Having personally experienced suffering, he has empathy with pain in the world. It's unlikely he will ever be a doctor, lawyer, or executive manager, but he already is a first-class human being.

### Spiritual journey

Kevin has an appreciation of the difference between work and vocation. Work is the job he carries out at the nursing home, folding and distributing laundry. It can be boring and tiring. But when Kevin remembers to look upon it as a service to God and humankind, it becomes a vocation. Then he sees it as the experience of sharing work with his housemates, and offering his presence to the residents and staff at the nursing home.

Carolyn Gratton speaks of a "personal vocational hunger" that, below the level of rational awareness, moves us to pursue our dream. "The vocation of every human person is to live in a covenant relationship of intimacy with God," she says.[1] Work becomes a vocation when we commit our time and effort in the service of God, for the needs of humankind and the care of the earth.

Throughout our lives, we are called to grow spiritually and become holy. To be holy is to be whole, appreciating and nurturing body, mind and spirit. In the words of Father Ron Rolheiser,

It's too simple to think that sanctity is merely a question of the "spiritual person" inside us triumphing over the person inside of us who loves this world, or over the child in us who is still given over to daydreaming. Wholeness means somehow making a whole, a harmony, out of all these different persons.... To be human is to be pathologically complex. But that points to our richness, not poverty, and suggests that all our different parts are important to the spiritual journey.[2]

In becoming whole and wholesome, we learn to recognize truth and respond to the beauty in all created things. Above all, we become increasingly aware of the loving presence of God. St. Bonaventure expresses the Franciscan awareness of God's presence in all of creation: "The physical universe and the soul of man are seen as mirrors reflecting God, and as rungs in a ladder leading to God."[3]

Thérèse of Lisieux believed that what pleases God most

is to see me love my littleness and my poverty, it is the blind hope I have in his mercy.... In other words, to become a saint, there is no need at all to feel great desires in one's heart. At Gethsemane, Jesus begged his Father to take away the chalice of suffering that awaited him. What does the Lord ask us to do? To recognize our radical powerlessness to attain true love by our own efforts and to expect everything from him.[4]

In wanting to draw souls to God, Thérèse, a Carmelite, reassures us of God's unconditional love and mercy despite our own spiritual deficits. Franciscan spirituality also honours the littleness of humankind and the incomprehensible love of God. In Francis' writings, the saint "slips inadvertently from references to the Spirit of God to the spirit of the human person. He perceives the dignity of the human personality, which could become the transparent expression of the divine presence."[5] His loving ministry to the lepers continued into the last years of his life, when he was seriously ill and nearly blind. Francis insisted that his followers, too, carry out dedicated care of the poor and afflicted.

Researchers studying forgiveness and resentment among institutionalized persons with disabilities found these individuals to be surprisingly forgiving, resentment-free and hopeful. In their relationship with God, "none experienced resentment towards God because of their disability, [and] in fact, some increased their faith in God and found God to be a great help in coping with disability." Likewise, even those who had been abandoned by their families or visited rarely expressed very little resentment. "They looked forward to any visit from a family member and most often considered the other patients and sometimes staff to be like family." Only towards the disability itself, whether it was developmental or caused by illness or accident, did they indicate some resentment. They said they wanted to be able-bodied like everyone else. Despite this latter regret, the majority of the disabled persons "demonstrated a hopeful attitude."[6]

We sometimes overlook the reality that the poor and afflicted experience the same quest for meaning in their lives that the less afflicted do. As well as being able to recognize in themselves the *radical powerlessness* that Thérèse admires, they also possess the great dignity of personhood extolled by Francis.

In their littleness, they are attuned to the Spirit of God, which guides us all in our quest to God. Francis and Clare, in *their* quest for meaning, believed that the gospel was meant to become our way of life. This is why the Secular Franciscan Rule instructs us to live our lives going from gospel to life and life to gospel. "Walking the way of the Gospel, we learn to sense the Spirit who makes our lives fruitful and creative, and this inner sense of the Spirit is a most sure guide for our journey."[7]

Our longing for God and God's invitation to us are integral to our being. We are drawn towards the Creator through our yearning for love, wisdom, justice and truth. As well, the beauty and workings of creation demand human interaction. Our guides are the Word of God and community spirit. Community is an essential element in spiritual development. Jesus tells us that where two or three are gathered, he is there. He instructs us to gather as community, reminding us that, however much we value our privacy, we need other people. It has always been a fundamental Franciscan conviction, says Frances Teresa, "that the Spirit speaks to the group when they are all together, listening to the Spirit and each other. The ideal is always consensus."[8]

Franciscan spirituality was created out of four things: Francis' total obedience to Christ, his prayer at all times, his desire to suffer with Christ, and his love of nature in all its forms.[9] To incorporate this spirituality into our lives, we strive to walk the gospel, live each day as a prayer offering to God, embrace all people as we would Jesus, and respect Mother Earth.

Regardless of the degree of our limitations, we seek meaning in our lives, our relationships, our work and our world. It is holy and wholesome to pursue a lifelong quest for meaning, and to encourage others on this quest.

In the process of becoming whole, we grow increasingly aware of truth, beauty and the loving presence of God in all of creation. In our quest for meaning, we reach for the Franciscan awareness of the physical universe and the soul of each individual as a mirror reflecting God.

# 11

# Going Home

**From Kevin's journal: Days 21 and 22**

*Day 21 – August 6, 1992 – Woodstock, Vermont*

"You slept very well last night, Kevin," I say.

"The tape was very relaxing," he explains. "The music was beautiful and there were sounds of birds and water and some other sounds. What are we doing today?"

"We'll be seeing some lovely scenery as we drive through New Hampshire and Vermont."

"I'm sad that we have only two more nights."

"I'm kind of sad too. But we're having such a terrific holiday, aren't we! And you're going on another holiday with St. Francis Advocates. That's something to look forward to."

"It will be okay. I really would prefer to live with you. Why don't we have a place like this motel and I could help you run it?"

"It's an interesting thought," I agree.

"We would be very happy here."

We set out again, and soon stop at an antique barn. "I see a pin I like," types Kevin.

"It has an Italian flag and an American flag," notes the owner. "It seems to be the Italian American Association. Here's another one from a New Hampshire ski resort."

"I liked the first one," decides Kevin.

"Fine. We'll buy it," says his dad.

Jim then strikes up a conversation with a couple who are also browsing in the barn. "I don't like Dad talking about me," types Kevin.

"Kevin, those people are retired teachers and they were very impressed with your computer. Dad's telling them how smart you are."

"That's good, but I still don't like it."

"Isn't it better that they think you're smart than think you don't know anything?" I ask.

"Yes. It's much better," Kevin admits.

Farther along, we stop at a New Hampshire camp store, and Jim goes in for supplies. He comes out and reports, "They have nice pins in there for Maine, New Hampshire and Vermont."

"Why don't you get all three?" I suggest.

"I'm happy Dad found the pins," says Kevin. Jay Jay, the voiceless mannequin, is now wearing all the pins we've been collecting. "When are we stopping for coffee?" asks Kevin.

"As soon as we find some," I reply. "You're doing so well today, Kev!"

But as we wander through another mall, Jim has a negative report. "I'm afraid Kevin had a slip."

"Well, Kevin, that's too bad," I sigh.

"It's not good," Kevin agrees.

"We want to make a few more stops. Can you handle it?"

"OK. As long as you don't waste time. Will I get coffee?"

"We'll see."

At another shopping stop, Kevin declares, "This is boring. Do I get coffee?"

"Yes. You've done well. Do you remember when we used to go camping?"

"It was wonderful. We were such a happy family then. We boys had lots of fun being together."

"I remember lots of fights," says Jim.

"Yes. But as far as I can tell, we loved each other," says Kevin. "Fighting is just what brothers do."

Later, we sit in another restaurant. "I'm starving," says Kevin. "Please can I have what Dad is having?"

"He's having the manicotti," I tell him.

"The manicotti will be great. I'm happy that we've had a great day even though I ate a butt. It seems that Dad is in a good mood. Dad certainly has a curious mind. He's always asking questions or walking about checking things out."

"Like plants?" asks Jim.

"He's always been like this," continues Kevin. "Even when we were children."

"Is that okay?" I ask.

"Yes. But it sometimes can be embarrassing for us. It seems I'm not as hungry as I thought."

"That's all right," says Jim. "We'll ask the waitress to put it in a box and you can eat it later."

"What's taking so long?" asks Kevin as we wait for credit card processing.

"They're probably doing a check to see if Dad's credit card is good," I explain.

"What would happen if it wasn't good?"

"We'd have to pay cash," explains Jim.

"That would be embarrassing," says Kevin, and adds with relief, as the waitress arrives with the receipt, "Good. It was accepted."

Day 22 – August 7, 1992 – Canandaigua, New York

"I'm sad that this is our last night on holidays," said Kevin the next day.

"We'll have to make this a really pleasant day," I said.

"Yes. We will try. Where are we going?"

"We'll travel through New York State and maybe look at microwave ovens since ours has died."

"As far as I can tell, that's okay. We need a microwave at home. As far as I can tell, I'll be having a good time soon with St. Francis Advocates."

"Yes, it should be a very nice holiday."

"As far as I can tell, I'm looking forward to school. As far as I can tell, I will have you facilitating."

"Probably," I say.

"That will be great. I plan to do well in school."

For a couple of days, we have been unable to reach our youngest son, Joel, who is minding things at home. After we make another futile attempt to phone him from a restaurant in Woodstock, New York, Kevin asks, "Are you worried about Joel?"

"I *would* feel better if we could get him on the phone," I admit.

"Perhaps he's working at St. Francis House," says Kevin.

Finally Jim emerges from a phone booth with good news. "I talked to Liz at St. Francis Advocates and she talked to Joel yesterday," says Jim. "Joel told her to expect Kevin tomorrow."

"As far as I can tell, Joel is okay. Liz said he's fine," says Kevin with relief. "Are we leaving the States today?"

"No. Not until tomorrow," I say.

"That's good."

Sometime later, we enjoy a restaurant lunch with an attentive waitress. After we refuse a second coffee refill from her, Kevin protests, "I would have liked more coffee."

"We've all had two cups with breakfast plus one at the motel. We mustn't overdo it," I say.

"That seems unnecessary."

"That's already one more than I'm supposed to have." And it certainly is more than Kevin needs to become anxious and agitated.

"That's too bad," types Kevin.

"What would you like for dinner?" I ask Kevin later, in a Chinese restaurant in Madison, New York.

"I want just what you have."

"We'll start with an egg roll. Do you want Chinese tea or coffee?"

"Coffee, because I have been exceptionally good."

"You certainly have. Do you think the smoke stick is a helpful reminder?"

"Yes. It's made me more aware about avoiding butts. I think I'm winning at last."

Later, Jim says to Kevin, "You should have listened to me about the Chinese tea. Then you would have refills, too."

"Dad should have told me that I didn't get refills of coffee," complains Kevin.

"Never mind. Have some tea. Break open your fortune cookie and see what it says."

"Simplicity is the sign of a good character," reads Kevin.

"Not quite. Take another look," I prompt.

"Simplicity of character is the result of profound thought."

"You left out a word."

"Natural."

"That's it. Simplicity of character is the natural result of profound thought."

"That describes you quite well, Kevin," says Jim. "You have lots of profound thoughts."

"Where is your fortune?" I ask later.

"I ate it."

"The paper?"

"Yes."

"Was it good?"

"Not really, but I thought it was part of the cookie."

"Not to worry. Those cookies are rather tasteless. It's hard to tell the difference between the cookie and the paper," I say.

Following dinner, we begin to search for a motel room. We drive through many towns, unable to find a vacancy. Finally, at a country place, Jim enters the inn's office just ahead of another family. Darkness has already fallen.

"Let's hope this motel has a room, Kevin," I say as we sit wearily in our car.

"I hope so. We might not find one for hours," types Kevin.

As it turns out, we obtain the last spot and watch the other family drive off into the night.

Once inside, Jim asks, "Shall I order a pizza? Are you hungry, Kevin?"

"I sure am. I thought you were going to let me starve."

"I was," teases his father.

"That's terrible. After all, this is the last day of my special holiday with you."

"How did you feel when we got the last motel room?" I ask Kevin as we wait for the pizza to arrive.

"I felt relieved for us, but I felt sorry for those other people. They must have been tired and discouraged. I hope they've found a spot by now."

"I hope so, too," I say.

"I'm a happy person," he then types. "We've had a great holiday and this is going to be an exciting year. I'm doing real subjects in school and my first book is finished."

Jim says, "Since tomorrow is the last day of our special holiday and you've had no butts today, I think we should stop at Niagara Falls."

"Great. It will be a great conclusion to our trip."

"Do you remember being there before?"

"As far as I can tell, I've seen it several times. I've been there with you and my brothers a few times, and I've been there with St. Francis Advocates once and with a school class once."

"Have you?" asks Jim. "You've got a good memory, Kevin."

## Belonging to family

In belonging to family, we each belong to a special place called home. Our need for this belonging is soul deep. Jean Vanier has said that a person cannot have two homes. I have come to believe that this is true. There is that one particular place that tugs at our hearts.

People living in the residences operated by St. Francis Advocates either have regular contact with their families or they've come from institutions and have little or no family interaction. Those with involved families seem always eager to "go home." While it is sometimes troublesome to residence dynamics, the desire to go home is healthy and wholesome. All of us, as long as our parents live, and no matter what our age, call the place where we were raised "home."

People from institutions, on the other hand, seem to adjust more readily to residential life. The new people in their lives soon become family to them. But as one residential counsellor recently told me, they always have a hole in their heart. There remains some deep longing within them, some primal need for love and belonging. They cling to visitors, even strangers, demanding the affection and attention that they've missed along the way.

When we are away from home, for business, pleasure or calling, we are grounded by the fact that somewhere we do have a home. Henri Nouwen says that everyone who returns from afar is "looking for someone waiting for him at the station or the airport. Everyone wants to tell his story and share his moments of pain and exhilaration with someone who stayed home, waiting for him to come back."[1]

The need for belonging is in our nature. We are drawn to seek out family and friends. We identify with neighbours, community organizations, co-workers and parishioners. Kinship is a magnet within our souls.

When I asked Kevin if he was content with his life, he responded, "I want to spend private time with you and Dad just like I do now." Kevin was stating that yes, he was content as long as he could touch home base on a regular basis. In this same conversation, Kevin also broached the benefits of having extended family.

"After you're dead," he typed, " I want my brothers and their families to keep in close touch with me. I would like to travel with them sometimes, too, and go to visit them. They can visit me whenever they wish."

Jewish author Edith Hahn Beer writes of her need to be with other Jews at the end of the Second World War. In late 1946, while employed as a Judge in Brandenburg, Germany, she learned of a transit camp in the French zone where Jewish survivors were gathering. Edith visited the camp, hoping to find news about her mother. "Besides, it was around Rosh Hashanah," she says, "and I longed to be with Jews."[2]

We are most comfortable with people of our own belief system, our own faith. People with disabilities have the same need to be included in parish activities. Roman Catholic canon law acknowledges and accommodates this need – at least in principle.

"In accord with Canon 777.4, pastors are responsible to be as inclusive as possible in providing evangelization, catechetical formation and sacramental preparation for parishioners with disabilities," notes the United States Bishops' Guidelines on this topic.[3]

A welcoming church community must have more than a ramp or elevator for the physically disabled. It must be fully accepting of all people, a model of the mind of Jesus Christ. "A fully accessible parish reaches beyond mere physical accommodation to encompass the attitudes of all parishioners toward persons with disabilities."[4]

All who have been baptized have the right to be properly instructed to receive the sacraments of confirmation, eucharist and reconciliation. Even persons who do not seem mentally competent are to be encouraged to receive the Holy Spirit in the sacrament of confirmation. If they do not know God as clearly as the rest of us think *we* do, God surely knows *them*.

The criterion for reception of holy communion is the same for all: the person is able to distinguish the body of Christ from ordinary food, "even if this recognition is evidenced through manner, gesture or reverential silence rather than verbally."

Moreover, "as long as the individual is capable of having a sense of contrition for having committed sin, even if he or she cannot describe the sin precisely in words, the person may receive sacramental absolution."[5] Those with profound mental disabilities can join the community in penitential services. The use of signs, writing, drawing and interpreters should be encouraged and made available.

An inviting church community makes sacraments available to all who are properly disposed to receive them. Cases of doubt are to be resolved in favour of the disabled person.

Once, when we were travelling, Kevin left a church greatly agitated. He was upset that the priest had placed the consecrated host on his tongue, rather than in his hand as other parishioners had received. "That priest thought I was stupid," he raged. Pastors and parish ministers must be sensitive to the feelings of everyone.

Kevin does not consider it at all exceptional that he has received the sacraments of baptism, eucharist, confirmation and reconciliation. He accepts it as his right as a member of the Church family. When we attend church, we are coming home to our Christian brothers and sisters.

Home is indeed where the heart is. Like love, home is an expansive entity. Home is the place of comfort that we seek at the end of the day. It may be the setting wherein we encounter our parish family. For the fortunate, home is not merely the place of origin, but the family homestead where there is unconditional acceptance.

For all of us, however, home is with God, not off somewhere beyond the stars, but wherever we are at any point in our existence.

## Spiritual journey

The longing within us for home comes from the bosom of God. It is the voice of God, calling us by name. It is the voice of Jesus calling us to come to him if we are weary and burdened. It is the voice of pilgrims past, reminding us that we shall not rest until we rest in God. Thus are we guided towards discovering ourselves and, more importantly, to finding God in ourselves.

When we reach this place, says Richard Rohr, "we will know and love ourselves, in spite of all the negative and opposing evidence. It is the spacious place of the soul. To live there is finally to be at home. This first and final home we carry with us all our lives."[6]

God is my destiny and God is with me in my soul, but I am still a human traveller. My restlessness is a reminder that I am still on pilgrimage. As pilgrims, it is our nature to experience ambivalence, forever longing to be somewhere else in order to become a better person. The dynamic of pilgrimage is the very dynamic of the human soul, notes Murray Bodo.

> We are both comfortable and uncomfortable with where we are. We are both comfortable and uncomfortable with who we are. We move between the two poles: We want to stay, we want to leave. We want to remain in a given state of being, and we want to move beyond that state.[7]

Kevin comes home often, and returns as often to his home with his two friends. He is usually happy to return to either place. Whenever he seems reluctant to leave us, I remind him that the coming workweek is a necessity for all of us. Life involves a rhythm of responsibilities and relaxation, time with friends and time with family. Kevin accepts this.

But lately he has been restless and discontented. Jim and I have agonized over this, hoping that contentment might be restored. We have had to acknowledge that when things are not quite right in our lives, it's an indication that change is needed. We have had to face up to the fact that Kevin is an intelligent, 35-year-old man. He has a right to be listened to and respected.

When I asked him what he would like if he were planning his own future, he replied, "I want to stay with the Daves sometimes and spend more time with you. But I still want my room in town kept private. No one should be in my room when I'm not there." Kevin is saying that he doesn't want his room to become a respite bed. Like everyone, Kevin wants ownership of his own personal space and belongings.

"How much time would you want to spend with us?" I asked.

"I would like to go home every other week for five days, plus on the Daves' weekends home, plus your holidays."

"It seems that you would be at home more than at your own place."

"That's what I want, to be home more than there."

Despite Kevin's living much of the time with the people of St. Francis Advocates, Jim and I continue to be actively involved in his life. Being a parent is a lifetime role for everyone, changing over time from one of total responsibility for one's children, to that of mentor, and finally to one of dependency on them. For parents of vulnerable children, however, there remains an urgency and immediacy that doesn't change with time. Our *attitude* towards the urgency and immediacy changes significantly, however.

As we live through the stages of our lives, our sense of reality expands. We become more attuned to our souls, the value of community, and the vastness of creation. We are increasingly drawn to simplicity, developing an inner core of resiliency and peace. Jean Vanier says that "it takes time to find the rhythm of life and the spiritual nourishment necessary to change our attitude and to welcome reality with serenity."[8]

Jim and I are genuinely glad that Kevin spends so much time with us. We treasure his company as much as he values ours. Our dogs are crazy with delight when he comes home, welcoming him with barks, whines and wags. One or other of the cats is often purring on his lap as he watches TV, or snoozing on his bed while he sleeps at night. To all appearances, Kevin neither returns their affection nor acknowledges their presence with any degree of enthusiasm. But the loving behaviour of the animals proves that something subliminal is certainly occurring.

On a Sunday morning in November 1999, we were lazily reading in bed, having attended Mass the previous evening. It was balmy for that time of year, and our bedroom window was open. Eric, our standard poodle, and Suzy, a border collie mix, had already been out for their morning run. Kevin was still sleeping. When the dogs began barking, we told them to be quiet. The barking persisted. Suddenly, both dogs leapt upon our bed, barking frantically while facing the door to the hall.

Cautiously, I got up and went down the hall to the kitchen. Initially, nothing seemed amiss. I peered into the family room which, joined to the living room, ran along the rear length of the house. Everything seemed strangely dim and hazy. Something was wrong but I couldn't quite place it. Just as I was about to wander into the family room, I glanced at the steel door joining the kitchen and garage. The door's white paint had turned completely black and wisps of smoke oozed through its outer edges. I stood there stunned, uncomprehending.

Then I knew. "Fire! Fire!" I screamed as I ran back towards the bedrooms. While Jim roused Kevin, I called 911. A rapid beeping sounded in my ear. Twice more, I called 911. Twice more, I heard the out-of-order beeping. Only moments had passed, but the house was now full of choking smoke. Hastily, we donned coats and boots over our pyjamas, leashed the dogs, and headed for the front door. Jim grabbed his wallet from the dresser. Bleu, our half-Siamese cat dashed through the door ahead of us. Sami, a timid Burmese, was nowhere to be found. As we stumbled through the door, the hall smoke alarm began to sound.

The hours that followed were a blur of activity and inertia. Fire trucks came from near and far. Cars parked and people stood along the road. St. Francis Advocates staff arrived and took Kevin back to his house. The fire chief told us that the entire attic had been ablaze before we even knew there was a fire. It was later determined that the fire had begun in the crawlspace under the family room (perhaps from wiring gnawed by voles or field mice), spread from there to the garage and thence to the attic. After that, the fire swept rapidly along the length of the house between roof and ceiling. The house was destroyed, with only the east walls left partially intact.

As the fire raged, I asked the firefighters to save Sami and my computer from the master bedroom. The novel I was writing was on my computer, and all my other writing was undoubtedly burning with the rest of our belongings. Jim sent me across the road with the dogs, where I sat on a neighbour's porch watching flames and black smoke devour our house. Our locked motor home, parked beside the garage could not be moved because its keys were in the fiery garage. Suddenly, the firefighters were backing up and ordering everyone out of the way. Then, in a dramatic explosion of flame, the motor home too was gone.

Only later would I contemplate the disappearance of cherished possessions collected item by item over 36 years. Through the years, we had accumulated antique and oriental furniture, some of the pieces unique. We also had limited-edition prints and hundreds of books and tapes. Then there were the musical instruments: a Yamaha grand piano, an old Baldwin church organ, Jim's Ovation and Yamaki guitars, the children's violins in various sizes, cymbals, triangles, castanets, and other rhythm instruments from my studio. All gone.

By far the most distressing was the loss of personal family treasures: photo albums, little gifts handmade or carefully chosen by the children in their growing-up years, scrapbooks, keepsakes that had belonged to my mother and grandmothers, a beautiful oval table once owned by Jim's grandmother.

Late in the day, the firefighters dared to enter the smouldering building. They retrieved a few damaged pieces of antique furniture and some china. Then they pushed through to the bedroom area and emerged with my computer and a soggy, sooty, slightly-scorched but living and breathing Sami! Also redeemed from the bedrooms was a filing cabinet containing our sons' baby books and some school mementoes, plus a dresser drawer of unsorted photos and negatives.

The house was then sealed off with yellow tape while inspectors combed it over the next two days. Then we were presented with a small box from the bedroom that had been Kevin's. It contained binders of letters and records pertaining to Kevin's history. One sooty binder contained the typed pages of Kevin's journal, his "book," painstakingly created during the summer of 1992 on our trip to the east.

For a month Jim and I stayed in a motel suite with the cats while the dogs were boarded at a kennel. Seeing our homelessness as an opportunity to make some life changes, we delayed rebuilding and moved into a rented farmhouse near Watford. Should we move north to be near our aging parents, we wondered? Should we retire to a cottage on the water? Might we work at a Franciscan retreat house? How would Kevin fit into any of this? Over the next several months, we investigated many options.

During this time, we experienced the generosity of a caring community. People stopped by with food and condolences. Family members maintained regular contact. Parishioners, friends and Franciscans from all over supported us with prayer and messages of encouragement. Their compassionate care sustained us in a powerful way. Although we certainly felt a sense of loss and displacement, we did not mourn the absence of our beautiful things. Even when we learned that our insurance did not begin to cover the contents of our house, we were accepting.

Three events from those early weeks remain with me as symbols of Christian spirituality: a tiny crèche, an anonymous donation, and a story.

The Wyoming Catholic Women's League dropped off a porcelain crèche at the motel so that we'd have a Christmas decoration for the season. I was touched by their kind gesture, and uplifted by the simplicity of the little white figurine. I keep it out year round now as a reminder of the love of the humble Saviour and the strength of community.

Around the same time, we received in the mail an unsigned card containing a $50 bill. From this I learned first-hand the value of anonymity. It has had a lasting corrective effect on my attitude towards people. Whenever I feel annoyance or an uncharitable thought towards someone, I then think, "What if this person is the one who anonymously sent us the money?" This thought immediately brings me back to gospel values. In seeing the donor in every face, I more clearly see Jesus in every face.

The third event was a story used in a homily by our pastor, Father Dan Vere. A retired couple had distributed their belongings among their children in order to move into a small cottage. Sometime after that, a fire destroyed the cottage and everything in it. "We have lost everything!" the woman wept. "No, we haven't," said her husband. "We still have everything we gave away." I mulled this over at length. Our earthly possessions, even the people we hold dear, are not ours to keep. Sooner or later we have to let them go. The consolation comes in the reality of the ever-present kingdom, and the continuum of our journey to God and with God.

The kingdom is present when God takes up his dwelling among us, says Murray Bodo, "and, as Francis reads the Gospel, God takes up his dwelling only when we are poor in spirit. It is not what we do that brings about the Kingdom, but what we embrace that God might dwell among us."[9]

Being poor in spirit is a constant process of becoming. The house fire enabled Jim and me to rebuild a simpler lifestyle. While we lived in the motel and then in the rented farmhouse, we found ourselves becoming increasingly content with a life of simplicity. We discovered the freedom of owning little. We wondered how we had become so materialistic, accumulating pretty things just to look at and touch. We were becoming familiar with Franciscan simplicity and poverty as never before.

One day while Francis was praying, writes Bodo, God spoke to his heart.

> Oh, Francis, if you want to know my will, you will have to hate and detest everything which till this moment you have loved and longed to make your own. And once you begin to do this, everything that previously seemed sweet and pleasant to you will become bitter and unbearable; and the things you once shuddered over will bring you great sweetness and you will be at peace.[10]

In coming face to face with a simpler version of home, we experienced God's sweetness and peace. We realized, too, that home can be wherever one dwells.

Jim and I avoided rebuilding for three years, but during our time of self-imposed exile, we gradually felt called back to our old place. Jim missed his gardens. Kevin needed his own space, as did our visiting children and grandchildren. And so we returned to our property, a serene five acres in the country outside the pleasant town of Petrolia. The house we built is smaller than the previous one. The furnishings are comfortable but simpler than those we had before. Still, our lifestyle is luxurious when rated against world standards.

It takes prayer to continue seeking the gospel vision of home. It takes determination to live out the gospel mission. In her *Testament*, Clare of Assisi exhorts all her sisters, those afar and those near, those present and those to come,

> to strive always to imitate the way of holy simplicity, humility, and poverty and to preserve the integrity of our holy manner of life.... Loving one another with the charity of Christ, let the love you have in your hearts be shown outwardly in your deeds so that, compelled by such an example, the sisters may always grow in love of God and in charity for one another.[11]

It is the longing of every person to be loved through a physical presence, an outward expression of the love in our hearts. Going home, wherever that is, be it humble or grand, provides a place of communion and acceptance essential to human existence.

# 12

# The Advocates

**From Kevin's journal: August 22, 1992**

This is the first time Kevin has been home since our trip to Nova Scotia. He has just returned from a vacation with the people he lives and works with at St. Francis House in Petrolia.

Today after I pick him up at his house in town, we drive to our family home in the country. "I'm happy to be home," he types.

"We're happy to see you," I reply. "How was your holiday with St. Francis Advocates?"

"It was great."

"What did you do?"

"I was with the St. Francis Advocates guys at a cottage in Port Elgin."

"Sounds like you had a good time."

"Yes. We had campfires and lots perhaps fun. Are you coming to school with me?" Kevin has done one of his abrupt topic changes because he is feeling anxious about the start of school. For the first time ever, he is going to be in a regular high school classroom. I plan to accompany him for a while until a teaching assistant feels comfortable facilitating with him.

"Yes, on Mondays and Fridays. How are you doing with butts?" I guess I can change the subject rather quickly, too.

"As far as I can tell, I'm doing very well."

"How many butts did you eat?" I ask.

"Sometimes none."

"What was the most you ate?"

"As far as I can tell, three."

"It's really important that you don't eat *any* at school." I have anxiety, too. It is important to our credibility with facilitated communication that Kevin performs appropriately. Kevin is aware of my concern.

"Yes. I want them to know how smart I am."

"I fixed Jay Jay for you," I say, suddenly remembering his old friend. "I had to do plastic surgery on his hand and foot. What do you think?"

"You did a great job." Kevin smilingly puts Jay Jay on his lap. Jay Jay is still wearing some of the collector pins we acquired on our trip.

"What do you want to do with him?" I ask.

"I want to take him back with me, and next year when we go on our holiday, I want to take him with us on the trip."

## 1990 – The Official Open House of St. Francis Advocates

The official opening of St. Francis House took place on October 5, 1990, one year after the first residents moved in. Our pastor, Father Frank White, blessed the home and a crucifix that had been donated in the memory of a deceased friend and attorney, Ray Wyrzykowski.

The Ministry of Housing and the Ministry of Community and Social Services sent greetings.[1] The provincial government sent a representative, as did the County of Lambton and local municipalities. Due to a change in government, our faithful supporter, David Smith, the previous Member of Parliament for Lambton, was no longer in office.

The media were well represented; I had already given an early-morning radio interview. Friends, families and neighbours gathered for the occasion, and Secular Franciscans came from several Ontario fraternities. Of course, board members and staff were out in full force, all of us moved and delighted by the atmosphere of support and celebration.

The occupants of the officially opened house welcomed their many guests graciously, and joined in the festivities. Visitors commented on the cheerfulness and peace that pervaded the home's atmosphere. One of our special guests was Temple Grandin, from Colorado, who would be our keynote speaker during the evening's annual meeting.[2]

I had driven to the Detroit airport on the previous day to meet Temple and deliver her to a Petrolia bed and breakfast. On the drive home from Detroit, I had the privilege of talking with this remarkable woman. Temple, who calls herself a "recovered autistic," has a Ph.D. in animal science and is an internationally recognized expert on animal behaviour and livestock facility design.

Throughout her talk that evening, I kept watching Kevin, who remained raptly attentive. Only later would I learn that he was indeed clinging to her every word, joyful that a person with autism had risen above her difficulties. A couple of years later, Kevin and I had the following conversation:

"When Temple Grandin spoke at the St. Francis Open House, how much of what she said did you understand?"

"I understood everything she said. She talked about the time she was in her aunt's barn and her aunt allowed her to use the cattle squeezer."

"Did she enjoy it?"

"Yes, she liked it very much. It made her calm."

"What does she do for a living?"

"She designs special equipment for farmers like ramps for animals who are being killed."

"What's special about these ramps?"

"They go around in circles, so the animals don't realize they will soon be dead."

"What did she say about being autistic?"

"She said it made her not like to be touched or wear clothes."

"Do you remember what she said things felt like against her skin?"

"Sandpaper," said Kevin.

"That's right. Did she have other problems?" I asked.

"She was reasonably normal, but she was distracted by noises and people moving around in the hall." On the drive to Petrolia, the squeaking of one of my car's windshield wipers as we drove through the rain had also disturbed her. Temple had repeatedly asked me if I couldn't make it stop.

"Do you remember one of the noises that distracted her in the hall that night?"

"The telephone," said Kevin.

Temple had, in fact, found an intermittently ringing telephone outside the hall quite bothersome. "Do you share any of her difficulties?" I asked.

"I don't like being touched, and I don't like loud people."

"You prefer when people speak softly to you?"

"Yes. I wish Dad would not shout so much."

"Dad has hearing loss and he keeps losing his hearing aid, so he doesn't realize how loud he sometimes is."

"That's terrible. Can anything be done about it?"

"If he goes to a clinic, they can make him a new hearing aid that will help him hear better."

"Then he should go soon."

## St. Francis Advocates Today

St. Francis Advocates operates five residential homes in Lambton County, and has started several other initiatives. The original farm residence is now known as St. Francis Farm. The other four houses are in Thedford, Port Franks, Forest and Petrolia. The Social Services ministry is urging them to start up other residences to accommodate residents from remaining institutions, which will close in the next few years. Kevin and two other young men have moved from the farm to a smaller house in the town of Petrolia. Each has his own room, and Kevin, who chose the smallest bedroom, has a private area downstairs for his computer, music and puzzles.

St. Francis Advocates runs a Supported Independent Living program to assist individuals living on their own in their communities. People with autism or other related disabilities receive help with money management, health and welfare, life skills development, and connecting with services within the community.

The Employment Services and Options program is comprised of academic programming, work experiences and community opportunities for people residing with St. Francis Advocates. The program offers integration within their community.

If requested by an agency or family, St. Francis Advocates will assist individuals and families to obtain supports and services available in their communities. The Community Supports program is funded through special contracts with the Ministry of Community, Family, and Children's Services (formerly the Ministry of Community and Social Services).

A Summer Day Program for adolescents and young adults operates out of St. Francis Farm during July and August. Young people from the area participate in recreational activities, social interaction, work skills training, life skills training and academics.

Stepping Stones is a collaborative planning service of St. Francis Advocates and the Family Network Group that is designed to assist young adults coming out of the education system. The initiative provides person-directed planning, goal setting, time-limited paid supports, and transition support.

St. Francis Advocates continues to live out its mandate to serve individuals with autism spectrum disorder and their families. It maintains the aspirations of its founding members to be forward thinking in areas of research, ongoing education, social and communication skills development, and the promotion of independence.

Most importantly, St. Francis Advocates recognizes that each person, as a child of God, has an innate dignity, along with physical, emotional and spiritual needs. To be whole, each person must have love, respect and full participation in decisions concerning his or her well-being.

It is now fifteen years since Kevin became the first resident of St. Francis Farm, and the first individual to benefit from the ministry of St. Francis Advocates. Both he and the organization are maturing nicely.

Through these years, he has attended high school, taken adult education courses, and audited courses at St. Peter's Seminary. He has been involved in work placements, including ones at a grocery store, high school library, and nursing home. St. Francis Advocates is always open to his changing needs and goals.

Remarkably, a few of the original staff, some board members, and all of the management personnel are still with us. Although keeping everything running smoothly can be a human resources challenge, the overall atmosphere remains relaxed and friendly. The spirit of Francis prevails.

To say that I am proud of the people who comprise St. Francis Advocates would be an understatement. Those who work with vulnerable individuals exhibit gospel poverty in their devotion to the well-being of the voiceless. Francis of Assisi showed us a way of solidarity with wounded people. In choosing to share our lives with these broken ones, we take upon ourselves their helplessness and failures. Like Francis, we become willing to be fools for Christ.

## Spiritual journey

Francis taught us a way of love, says Bodo,

that leaves us entirely poor in our helplessness and dependence on God.... Life among the lepers is always madness to those for whom respectability is holiness and safety is the norm. True poverty of spirit is never in safety but in the risk of looking for God where God said he was to be found, among the least of his brothers and sisters.[3]

When we assume solidarity with vulnerable people, we join the poor-in-spirit club. We find joy in small accomplishments, innocent laughter, silent closeness. We are inspired by their courage, generosity and humility. We also take on the frustrations, humiliation, ridicule and sorrow that are integral to their lives.

The number of people you can personally embrace is limited, says Bodo, because of the emotional drain of loving those who are broken. Moreover,

> you are caught up in the dilemma of closeness and distance, problems of what kind of intimacy is proper and what is not, something you do not have to face if you love humanity en masse but never get close enough to become involved with the pain of another.[4]

Holocaust survivor Elie Wiesel said that the opposite of love is not hate but indifference. Hate is readily recognized as evil, but indifference can, and does, pass unnoticed. The people of St. Francis Advocates are anything but indifferent. They are open to change, yet properly cautious. They are willing to try traditional treatments as well as alternative therapies. They encourage home visits and holidays with family members wherever possible. It is not unusual for them to include individuals from their programs in their own family celebrations, and to have them for overnight home visits.

Franciscan philosopher John Duns Scotus holds a central position among Franciscan thinkers for two reasons:

> first, he articulates philosophically the insight of St. Francis on the beauty of creation as a gift from God and, second, he develops and enhances the traditional Franciscan preference for love over knowledge as key to the human journey toward union with God.[5]

Within St. Francis Advocates, love is lived out as the key to the human journey to God. This was clearly felt with the approaching death of Thomas, who came to St. Francis Farm from an institution after Kevin and the Daves had moved into town. He had no known family, no folks who claimed he belonged to them. Like many developmentally challenged people, Thomas's physical health was fragile. In time, his condition deteriorated further, until he could barely shuffle about on his painfully swollen legs and he had difficulty breathing.

When Thomas was hospitalized for the last time, it was St. Francis Advocates staff who sat at his bedside, holding his hand, and reassuring him that he was not alone as Sister Death drew near. The entire Farm assembled to lovingly plan every detail of his funeral. Father Michael O'Brien, the priest from Alvinston where Thomas had attended Mass whenever he was able, said he felt greatly honoured to be invited to preside.

Thomas's funeral was as beautiful as any funeral ever held. The entire population of St. Francis Advocates was in attendance to celebrate his place in our hearts, and to mourn his passing. It was the essence of Franciscanism: the poverty of Thomas, the plainness of his coffin, the choice of prayers and music, the unpretentiousness of the participants, the uplifting words of the priest. Later, we stood under umbrellas in the rain for the graveside liturgy, and gathered afterwards at the farm to share food and memories. The simple marker at Thomas's grave was soon replaced with a granite monument donated by the Knights of Columbus, and erected at no cost by the local monument dealer.

An important opportunity to celebrate together takes place at the annual Christmas party. The entire St. Francis Advocates community, along with families and friends, comes to the festivities. Gifts are distributed by a Santa whose other role is father to a staff person. Everyone participates in dinner, dancing and noisy merriment.

Of course, there are many other events and outings – bowling, swimming, camping, concerts, movies, picnics and trips. Everyone who participates is teacher and student, giver and receiver. Jesus spent his time with people who had to struggle to belong. Francis imitated him; in the St. Francis Advocates community, we have the opportunity to join their exalted company.

In this community of pilgrims, we are all healers, and we are all servants. Catherine Doherty, founder of the international Madonna House lay apostolate community, speaks of the pilgrims of Russia, who were sought out for their wisdom, holiness and healing. These men and women often left lives of luxury to live in secluded huts known as a *poustinias*. Their lives were a combination of contemplative prayer and community service. Doherty explains that a *poustinik* or hermit put aside his bible and meditation when someone needed help "because he is in the poustinia of his heart always, especially when serving his fellowmen."[6]

Those of us who struggle with prayer versus action can be heartened by her words. When we serve one another, we are at prayer in the poustinias of our hearts.

The people in the employ of St. Francis Advocates work *for* the persons who are vulnerable. Because the vulnerable are seldom in a position of power, and many cannot express their wishes, it's easy to forget who works for whom. Once when Kevin was complaining about his dependence on staff, I told him that he was their boss. I pointed out to him that the staff were paid by the Daves and him to assist with day-to-day living and to enrich their lives. Kevin was astonished by this information.

"You have the right to tell them when you're not happy about something, or if there's something they can do to help you," I told him.

"I do?" he asked.

"Yes, you do," I said. "And you can even have them fired if you're not pleased with their assistance. Is there anyone you think should be fired?"

"No. They all seem to be doing a good job," said Kevin. "Do the staff know about this?" He was still absorbing the possibilities.

"They should," I said, thinking back to my own nursing days, when patients had few rights (and certainly weren't told about the rights they had). It's a characteristic of us in the health and social service fields to sometimes overlook our serving roles and get a bit bossy. We forget that what *we* think is best for the patient (or client or resident) may not be what the individual wishes. In our zeal for proper procedure, we may ignore the individual's rights.

"I feel much better now that I know the staff are working for me," said Kevin. I made a mental note to mention this conversation to the Advocates management team. Staff members are dedicated and devoted to the individuals they assist. It is the individuals themselves who need to be reminded that they do have some power over their lives.

God places in all of us the desire to accomplish something meaningful. Bodo writes that "Francis, like any young man, wanted to do something with his life, become someone, make a contribution that would be uniquely his. He was constantly asking God to enlighten his mind and heart."[7] It's in our creative natures to want to contribute uniquely to our world. Possibly the greatest challenge for caregivers is to permit everyone – individual, staff, volunteer – to make decisions and have control.

Pastor and clinical psychologist Kenneth Haugk tells caregivers that their responsibility is "to prepare the ground for the Great Curegiver. Preparing the ground means doing the best possible job to create a therapeutic situation and then waiting on the Lord expectantly. It is God who provides emotional, mental, physical, and spiritual growth according to his will."[8] In other words, caregivers provide care; God provides growth.

Haugk points out that when caregivers rely on God for results, they free themselves from worry and false expectations. Instead, they "can concentrate on creating the best therapeutic situation for growth to occur: developing trust and communicating acceptance and love."[9] The St. Francis Advocates community strives for this ideal.

# 13

# Confronting Rejection and Loneliness

### After the journal

*September 26, 1994 — Petrolia*

It's a pleasant family gathering, and Kevin's brothers and their families are together, sharing memories and laughing. Suddenly, Kevin becomes agitated, jumping and demanding attention. I bring him his new Lite Writer computer, and he types, "I want coffee immediately, and I am displeased with you. So why are *you* happy?" He presses the TALK button and glares appropriately as the synthesizer voice expresses his annoyance.

"Should I be unhappy?" I query.

"No, but you should be more attentive to me."

"Are you jealous that I'm talking to Laurie?"

"Yes. I am your son."

"And she is my daughter," I say.

"No. She is married to my brother."

Conversation drifts to other topics. Kevin listens in on a story that his father is reading to Kevin's nieces, Melissa and Mary. It's a book called *A Promise Is a Promise*, by Michael Kusugak. Jim brought it home from school. It's the story of a young girl who, after disobeying her parents and fishing on the sea ice, has to use her wits to escape a creature that wants to keep her under the water.

"Did you like *A Promise Is a Promise*?" I ask.

"It was a terrible story to tell little girls, and I'm distressed that Dad would abuse children psychologically."

Overhearing Kevin's criticism on the Lite Writer's computer voice, Jim interjects, "The story is meant to teach children that it's dangerous to go out on the ice."

"That appears logical but I'm not convinced that it has merit."

"Who is in the picture on your bulletin board at St. Francis House?" asks Laurie, who had visited Kevin's house earlier in the day.

"It's a picture of James and some girl he once knew."

"Who do the staff think the girl in the picture is?" asks Laurie.

"I have no idea," says Kevin. "As far as I can tell, the staff think it's his wife but they're confused. It's time they knew the truth. I am eager to show off my family."

"Even me?" asks Laurie, alluding to his earlier complaint about my diverted attention.

"Yes, Kevin," I say. "You said you were jealous when I spoke to Laurie."

"That has nothing to do with the way I feel about her. It's only right that I want your attention when I have been neglected by you for so long."

"Do you feel I neglected you?" I ask.

"As far as I can tell, you did your best but you should have realized how unhappy I was in Toronto."

"I had no way of knowing how intelligent you were, or how reasonable you might be," I try to explain. "Your behaviour didn't indicate that. What could I have done differently?"

"You would have taken me home and nurtured me into health. I'm not really unhappy with you. I love you and know that you love me. As far as I can tell, you did a fairly good job with all your sons, including me, and you didn't neglect or abuse any of us. Is Laurie a social worker?"

"Yes, she is," I say.

"Does she think I was abused?" asks Kevin.

"Laurie, do you think Kevin was abused?" I ask my daughter-in-law.

"What do you think, Kevin?" inquires Laurie.

"I was sent away when I was only twelve and I was very lonely."

"Why do you think that happened?" asks Laurie.

"I was addicted to solvent sniffing, and my brothers didn't want my mother to spend all her time on me. They wanted me sent away," types Kevin.

"Did you hear them say that?" asks Laurie.

"Yes. They said they didn't want a brother like me."

"'A brother like you,' what does that mean? How did they want you to be different?" asks Laurie.

"They wanted me to be treated for my addiction so I could come back home."

Laurie: "Who wanted you to get treatment?"

"My parents and my brothers."

Laurie: "How did they help you?"

"They started the autistic association here and St. Francis Advocates so I could be close to them."

Laurie: "Was that a helpful decision for you?"

"Are you wanting to know if they took care of me?"

Laurie: "Well, why do you think they did what they did?"

"They had to think of the mental health of the family."

Laurie: "So, do you think they made a good decision?"

"My parents wanted to preserve the family, including me, and they loved all of us equally."

Laurie: "So, they did the best they could?"

"As far as I can tell, it's the truth. But it still hurt me because I couldn't tell them I was aware of everything that was said about me."

Laurie: "What things were said that upset you?"

"My brothers said they wished they didn't have a brother like me and I heard them say it."

Laurie: "How do you think things would be different if they had known you understood what they were saying?"

"They would have treated me intelligently. I would not have started solvent sniffing if I hadn't been isolated from everyone."

Laurie: "Did the sniffing help you cope?"

"Yes. I could escape into a nice feeling and forget that I was autistic."

Laurie: "How are you doing now with your addictions?"

"As far as I can tell, I'm much better, but I still feel sensory deprivation and like to sniff things."

Laurie: "Do you think your addiction is better?"

"Yes, it is better. But I need to sniff things."

Laurie: "Is there anything your brothers should do to help you?"

"Yes. They should apologize to me and tell me they recognize my pain and tell me they love me."

Laurie: "Do you want to go tell them that now?"

"You tell them for me what I told you. I want them to know how I feel. They should be more sensitive to my feelings."

Laurie: "I think it would be better if you told them. Your mom and I can be there with you."

"Why should I be the one doing all the seeking when they will not approach me with anything personal? They just kid around and pretend everything is fine."

Laurie: "I know it will be hard to do, but I still think it needs to come from you directly."

"I will write them a letter expressing my feelings. Thank you for listening and clarifying my thoughts. I really have not realized how angry I felt towards my brothers. I thought I was just angry at my mother."

Later, Kevin types, "Ask Dad if he is disappointed in me. Does he wish I wasn't here? Would he like a different son?"

"Kevin, of course I don't want a different son," says Jim. "I'm very proud of you."

"I'm glad that Dad snorted at my question," says Kevin. "I need a lot of reassurance right now. I feel very vulnerable. I need to be loved fiercely. I have to know that I won't ever be abandoned. I want to be always nearby and included in all family events. Why wasn't I at the Pearson Christmas this year?"

"We haven't had the Pearson Christmas yet," says Jim. "It's on December 19. We love you and try to include you in everything that's going on."

"I know all that. But when I need to talk to you, you aren't there and I have no way of communicating with you. Please buy me a deaf phone so I can phone you like my brothers can. Six hundred dollars is not much compared to the money you have spent on their university fees. I need your support and you are my father."

"We'll get you one for Christmas," promises Jim.

"That would be a great Christmas gift. Arden will get one for St. Francis House and you will only have to get one for the house. I expect you to care enough to do this for me. Good night. See you in the morning."

## Entering the Silence

We are all broken people seeking wholeness. Ever since our expulsion from Eden, we have tried to fill the void of discontent with power and various amusements. We chase after a dream of happiness that flutters before us like a beautiful but illusive fantasy. When we are spiritually inquisitive, we come to see that the closer we come to the perfection that Jesus calls us to, the more we experience joy and peace. But, as saints through the ages have reminded us, true happiness will be experienced only in eternity with God. And as saints have reminded us, periods of spiritual joy are interspersed with experiences of the desert or wasteland.

One such experience descended upon an entire town in late May 2000. A week before Jim and I were to leave with my parents on a motor home trip, my sister from Walkerton, Ontario, phoned to say that Mother was sick with a gastric bug. The whole town had it, Patti told me. The following day, Patti and my other sister, Bonnie, took Mother to the hospital. The Emergency department was full of people with similar symptoms: bloody diarrhea, vomiting, cramps and fever. They were all sent home and told to drink lots of water.

On the following day, Monday, Mother was placed in intensive care, and early Tuesday, I drove to Walkerton. Mother had already received the sacrament of the sick, and as we stood around, helpless witnesses to her suffering, she was intubated and flown by helicopter to London. Shortly after midnight, with her husband and children at her side, my mother died.

By this time, it was known that the cause of the illness was E. coli contamination in the municipal water supply. A boil-water advisory was issued, and bleach and bottled water were made available to everyone in town. Even with all the precautions, several visitors, Kevin and I among them, became ill during our few days in town before and after Mother's funeral. All in all, more than 2000 people became acutely ill; seven, including Mother, died. One of the other fatalities was the two-year-old child of a doctor from a nearby town who had sipped water in a Walkerton restaurant four days earlier. Several children and adults were left with chronic kidney and bowel conditions.

Despite their personal suffering, the townspeople brought food to my sister's house, and attended Mother's wake and funeral. They had several funerals to attend and many people to console. It was good they reached out, because apart from close relatives and media, outsiders shunned the town. One of my memories of Mother's wake is the smell of bleach on everyone's hands.

The Walkerton water situation dragged on publicly for four years: years of inquiries, interviews, meetings, phone calls and media coverage. The Ontario Provincial Police dutifully kept us abreast of court dates and the progress of their criminal investigation. An entire town, plus those connected to it, lived suspended lives. In January 2002, Justice Dennis O'Connor released the report on the public inquiry begun in October 2000. To no one's surprise, the tragedy was declared preventable, and blame was placed on government cuts, the ineptitude of the Environment Ministry, and the Koebel brothers' dishonesty and carelessness. In November 2004, Stan Koebel, former manager of Walkerton's Public Utilities Commission, was sentenced to one year in jail. Frank Koebel, Public Utilities Commission foreman, received a conditional sentence that included nine months of house arrest.

A year after his grandmother's death, Kevin wrote about the pain of his loss.

> My grandmother was one of the dearest people in my life. She loved me unconditionally and never made me feel different. I loved the way she teased me and smiled at me. She was always happy to see me. After she died, I was very sad, and angry that the Walkerton water killed her.
>
> As far as I can tell, she suffered terribly, and she didn't deserve that. I didn't have the chance to say goodbye to her. I wanted to touch her warm skin again, and feel her hugs. Why did such a terrible thing happen to my family? My poor grandfather is a broken man. He will never be happy again no matter how much we try. My life is lonely without my grandparents' joy.
>
> I want the Walkerton water situation to never happen again to innocent people. My grandmother should have lived much longer and spent more time with me. She should have died

a peaceful death at home, not with tubes stuck into her. I cannot stop being angry.

Vulnerable persons are especially anxious about losing the people they love. Because they tend to have a limited circle of friends, family is especially important to them. On top of this, persons with autism are prone to anxiety that feeds upon obsessive thoughts. And so, long after his grandmother's death, Kevin was still lamenting his loss. "I miss the love and attention Grandma Pearson gave to me," he said. "No one else acted so excited to see me. She was such an interesting part of my life. Every day I think about her and who she was."

In August 2002, Jim's mother died, as did my father in late November. Again we mourned. We struggled to move beyond our misery and place our trust in God's healing power.

The pain of loneliness and rejection are inescapable for earth's inhabitants. But so are peace and healing. Life is a journey, an adventure, an opportunity. Its paths are lined with joys and sorrows, twists and turns, ups and downs. We do not know what awaits us around the next bend, nor do we know the length of our journey on the planet.

But we do have grace sufficient for the journey. When we allow our wounds to enter into the silence of our beings, we know Jesus. We know peace.

"Am I my brother's keeper?" Cain asked God. The answer, of course, is yes. Despite the distances that separate many family members in today's world, we remain responsible for each other's well-being. Parents continue to hope that their sons and daughters will care for each other in some capacity throughout their lives.

People who have no remaining blood relationships still require family. Sometimes a caring community needs to intervene to provide support. It may be as simple as assisting someone with weekly grocery shopping, or as complex as organizing 24-hour-a-day care.

Autism causes cognitive idiosyncrasies that interfere with social interactions. Like other vulnerable people, those with autism struggle regularly with loneliness and the regret that they are different.

Referring to her autism, Temple Grandin acknowledges that she does not fit in with the social life of her community. Most of her social contacts are work-related. "My interests are factual and my recreational reading consists mostly of science and livestock publications," she says. "I have little interest in novels with complicated interpersonal relationships, because I am unable to remember the sequence of events. Detailed descriptions of new technologies in science fiction or descriptions of exotic places are much more interesting."[1] Grandin acknowledges her limitations and builds activities around her strengths.

Kevin, who is additionally handicapped by being mute, is likewise trying to build a meaningful life for himself. He shares our love of nature, hiking, camping and travelling. We therefore make an effort to insert as much of this into his life as possible. Kevin, Jim and I frequently spend time in our motor home nestled in the woods and, over the years, have travelled throughout Canada and the United States.

In the fall of 1996, the three of us enjoyed a five-week motor tour of France and Italy, with stopovers in Germany, Austria, Switzerland and Spain. Kevin especially enjoyed the spirituality of Assisi and Lourdes. Religion and spirituality add a dimension of strength, courage and joy to Kevin's life. He enjoys attending Mass with his housemates or with us, and also attends a weekly Christian Friendship gathering.

Lifelong education is as important to persons with disabilities as it is for everyone. A few months ago, Kevin acquired an updated voiced computer, a Dynavox. He will undoubtedly continue to benefit from advances in computer technology.

This past summer, Kevin began taking medication that has decreased his obsessive-compulsive tendencies. He no longer lies awake at night tormented by obsessive thoughts. Outbursts of angry frustration have become a thing of the past. Rested and more in control of his behaviours, Kevin is far less anxious and seldom depressed. He describes himself as "a different man."

And so we thank God for the blessings that continue to filter through our lives. We welcome the calling that has placed us amidst the vulnerable people in the family of God.

**Spiritual journey**

When we absorb our wounds into the fabric and silence of our souls, we become more compassionate and sensitive. We become graced through the suffering shared by all of humankind.

"The great challenge is living your wounds through instead of thinking them through," observes Henri Nouwen. "It is better to cry than to worry, better to feel your wounds deeply than to understand them, better to let them enter into your silence than to talk about them."[2]

Following my mother's funeral, I sank into an abyss of sadness totally unlike my serene acceptance of the house fire six months earlier. I relived Mother's death over and over in my mind. My sleep was disrupted by nightmares and hours of wakefulness. Sometimes I was consumed with guilt: guilt for not fulfilling a promise to Mother that she would have a peaceful death; guilt for not doing enough to ease her deathbed pain; guilt for not spending enough time with her while she was alive. Other times I was consumed with anger: anger against the public health unit for taking four days to issue a boil-water advisory, four days that may have cost my mother her life; anger against the provincial government and their obsession with cutbacks, cutbacks that led, among other things, to inadequate supervision of municipal water plants; anger against an inattentive town council that, for many years, allowed two men's carelessness to jeopardize the health of an entire community.

During this period, I kept praying even though I felt spiritually bereft. Gradually, the sadness lessened along with the guilt and anger. Then, for a long time, I remained in a state of spiritual lethargy, with no desire to write or sing or play the piano. I wondered when my creativity would return, knowing that it would. I sensed that now I was waiting purposefully.

Clinical psychologist Fredrica Halligan writes of a patient who came to realize that she was not in control of her spiritual life. "It became clear that her spiritual life had a path of its own and that she was being directed to wait.... So we waited and trusted. Her own spiritual process would emerge in its own way and its own time."[3]

Once we get past the trauma of loss and tragedy, we are able to proceed with renewed strength and peace. The earlier suffering is incorporated into our beings, and becomes part of who we are. We would not choose the bad experiences that enter our lives, but out of the darkness we see others with a new empathy and deeper compassion. We become persons of finer texture.

When people with disabilities experience the trauma of loss and tragedy, they too can be reminded that this is an inescapable part of being human. We can reassure them that these trials are only threads in the tapestry of our existence, and are, moreover, essential to personal growth and development. Then these vulnerable individuals can better accept that they are not alone in experiencing the pain of rejection, denials of affection, and lack of support, real and imagined, that occur in their lives.

"Grief is necessary," writes Jean Vanier.

It is like a pruning, a pruning to help us return to what really matters and to communion. We then no longer live in a world of dreams or by escaping into the future, and we are not dependent any more on what others think of us and on their admiration. There comes a time when we can no longer hide. We simply meet God in our poverty, and he calls us to enter into communion with him.[4]

Moreover, it is possible to survive suffering without understanding why it happened. Viktor Frankl helped save himself and other concentration camp prisoners from despair by finding meaning in suffering. Sometimes one cannot act upon a situation but can only accept one's fate. Seeing suffering in this way enabled the prisoners to take suffering upon themselves as a task. "Therefore, it was necessary to face up to the full amount of suffering, trying to keep moments of weakness and furtive tears to a minimum," writes Frankl. "But there was no need to be ashamed of tears, for tears bore witness that a man had the greatest of courage, the courage to suffer."[5]

People who are different, for whatever reason, develop early the courage to suffer. If they did not, they would go mad. Toddlers tantrum when they are unable to control their environment. If these same toddlers have disabilities, they will continue to be limited in their ability to control their lives. To overcome the inevitable frustrations and despair takes tremendous courage.

People who have developmental or physical disabilities are regularly exposed to the thoughtlessness of others. They courageously tolerate insults, ridicule, indifference, rejection and terrible loneliness. Their stoicism is often mistaken for lack of awareness. Their smiling faces conceal the woundedness of their hearts. Their eyes can only hint at the pain within.

It is only when we experience suffering ourselves that we can begin to relate to our suffering sisters and brothers. It is only when we acknowledge our own limitations, dependencies and loneliness that others can relate to us.

Francis showed us all that self-sufficiency is an illusion, notes Bodo.

> We all need one another and we need God in order to know that we do need one another. And once we embrace our basic dependence on God and interdependence on one another, once we face and articulate the deep fear that keeps us from acknowledging any kind of dependence, then true dialogue is possible, that freeing dialogue that gives us the independence we were so afraid of losing.[6]

This morning, as I was supervising Kevin's bath, I sang snatches of "Wind Beneath My Wings" to him. "I'm singing this song to you, Kevin," I told him, "because you are my hero. You're the bravest man I know."

His face lit up with such joy and gratitude that I turned away to hide my tears. How often has Kevin been complimented on his bravery? How often is anyone complimented for being courageous? Yet we all need to be recognized in this way, for Jesus himself taught us that it takes courage and grace to be fully human.

# 14

# Pilgrims' Process

**Pilgrimage to Europe: September–October 1996**

Since the earliest times, pilgrims have travelled to sacred places seeking healing, wholeness and help. They love to tread where holy feet have walked, and to experience what sainted senses might have enjoyed. By the time of Francis and Clare, pilgrimages to the holy sites of Rome, Compostela and Jerusalem were undertaken by many. Clare's mother made a pilgrimage to the Holy Land to pray for a safe pregnancy and delivery. During his life, Francis travelled to Rome, Syria, the Near East and the Holy Land. Part tourists, part mystics, modern pilgrims diligently photograph museum and shrine alike, while collecting souvenirs for those back home.

In September 1996, four years after the trip to Nova Scotia, Kevin, Jim and I set out on a five-week European pilgrimage that would include Rome, Assisi and Lourdes. We did not name a particular grace or healing, but we acknowledged that we were seeking something special for Kevin, as well as anything God might see fit to give *us*. Kevin was very excited. Months before our departure, we plotted out a route, leased a Renault, and reserved a few rooms at selected spots along the way. In our usual manner, we left the rest to chance.

We flew from Toronto to Paris, slept the first afternoon away, and later walked the evening streets of that romantic city. As we prepared for bed, I treated Kevin's feet for plantars warts – six on his left foot, and eight on the right! It was a wonder that he could walk, and incredible that he didn't complain. We spent three days in Paris, seeing the usual wonderful things – Eiffel Tower, Musée d'Orsay, Les Invalides and Napoleon's tomb, the Louvre, Sainte-Chapelle, Notre Dame Cathedral.

Over the next few days, we travelled through the beautiful countryside and quaint towns of France. We loved the rolling fields and the little farm communes, walled-in mini-towns with barns and houses. We were thrilled when the highways merged directly into the narrow streets of adorable stone villages. Everything in Europe is so wonderfully old and steeped in history. As we wandered through remote areas, heading for sights unknown, we were never lost because we had no set destination.

Switzerland surprised us with its modern architecture, an abrupt contrast to the ancient charm of France. Its towns and cities were pretty and ornate in the Swiss style. Vineyards had taller plants than those of France, lending a different appearance to agriculture. One small town featured a fantastic Roman amphitheatre from 2 AD as well as a castle museum. It was a day of very changeable weather – sun, rain, hail.

When we reached Zurich, we had difficulty finding a place to stay. It was not until after midnight that we found lodgings in another town. In the confusion, we missed our appointed call home to Joel. Such are the perils and inconveniences of pilgrimage and of life.

The next morning we set out on a beautiful drive past Swiss mountainsides patterned with dwellings, churches and pastures. The road passed through incredibly long tunnels.

Germany enchanted us with its rolling hills and large farms with houses attached to barns. As in Switzerland, brown cows with pretty faces and belled necks grazed placidly. We passed two roadside shrines, and stayed overnight at a small *gasthof*. The inn's dining room contained a corner shrine with crucifix, dried roses and candles. That night, Franciscans around the world would also pray before a crucifix, celebrating the death of Francis in a ritual known as Transitus. St. Francis of Assisi died on a Saturday evening, October 3, 1226, going forth joyfully to meet Sister Death.

The following day we headed for Dachau, pausing, as on every day, to pray the Liturgy of the Hours. On this particular day, spiritual nurturing turned out to be especially welcome. Dachau was stark, moving, sobering. I couldn't help but reflect on how Nazis had first euthanized their own disabled citizens – men, women and children – before extending their evil towards able-bodied Jews and others who displeased them. Picturing the starved, ragged people forced to share wooden bunks, far too few toilets, humiliation and degradation brought tears to our eyes. I felt, for the first time, that I was truly on pilgrimage, walking on ground sanctified by blood and tears. It was appropriate that it was October 4, feast of St. Francis.

We live in a world of good and evil. So did Francis. But Francis became so centred on God that nothing was a distraction, notes Bodo.

> Our greatest distractions come not from the beauty of the world but from the evil in the world and in the self which we have not yet faced, which we try to suppress or deny. The religious person who cannot accept the reality of evil normally sugars everything with piety and distances the self from evil by loving in generalities; loving the poor, all people, nature, creation, and so on.[1]

Francis was not afraid to face evil or to embrace his own evil and potential for evil.

We returned to Austria, spending the night at a pleasant *pension* in Salzburg, the birthplace of Mozart. Mozart began his career as the most gifted child in the history of music, composing before the age of five. As if in tribute, bells chimed the hours within the inn, and in the city, church bells rang through day and night. It seems appropriate to pause here to compare two little boys with different sets of extraordinary gifts: Wolfgang and Kevin. One child would amaze an adoring world with his unusual talents. The other would puzzle a bemused world with his unusual behaviours. Both children were isolated by the societies of their day for their exceptionalities.

On another day, Jim, Kevin and I attended Mass in a beautifully ornate church along the Danube. Worship lasted an hour and a half, and was somewhat difficult to follow. The priest delivered several brief talks in German, and children intermittently sang and clapped. After Mass, everyone was served bread and wine outside the church. We were told it was Thanksgiving.

Eventually, we found ourselves in magical Venice. Our hotel room abutted a canal where gondolas and motorized boats floated by. It was surreal! We tried to get Kevin to admire the barges delivering groceries beneath our window, but he stayed back in the room's interior, finding the water's proximity too alarming.

Kevin typed, "Venice is very nice, but not as I expected. It's not as spacious, and more shabby than I thought it would be."

Venice *is* a little worn and water damaged, but it's splendid nonetheless. We saw the Cathedral of San Marco, vast and old, with its painted ceilings and ancient tiled floors. We visited the Doge's Palace, gazing upon intricately painted ceilings, wonderful statues, detailed frescoes. The next morning, we wandered around Venice for the last time, marvelling at the activity hidden by ancient walls: schools, businesses, residences, most of which are out of sight. While taking the waterbus back to the car park, we caught glimpses of this secret life. Along the water's edges were trees, gardens and rear entrances to villas, convents and other establishments.

Next we drove along Italy's northeasterly coast, where dingy landscape soon gave way to lovely scenery. Hillsides were dotted with villages, castles and remote stone dwellings. The road was treacherous in places: narrow, winding and sporadically walled in stone. Signage was vague and puzzling, and we were frequently disoriented.

**Search for healing**

At last we reached our villa overlooking Florence, a convent guesthouse with a tranquil courtyard and halls with marble tiles and pillars. Calm like her surroundings, and speaking no English, a Franciscan sister led us to our rooms. We had explained by e-mail from Canada that Kevin required personal assistance. The nuns therefore assigned us two bedrooms – one for me and the second for Jim and Kevin – and a bathroom key. A privacy sign was then posted on the door to the nearest bath, which seemed to puzzle other guests, and made us a bit embarrassed.

The villa was truly lovely. From its lofty perch, the lights of Florence could be seen twinkling below. In planning our trip, we had selected places we would visit and places that, due to time restrictions, we could not. Sadly, Vienna and Florence had been eliminated.

Early the next morning, we headed for Rome by train, leaving our car at the Orvieto station. When we arrived at our *pensione* in Rome, we were greeted warmly in faltering English by Franciscan Sisters. In the evening we walked to nearby St. Peter's Square and admired the massive columns there. Although the Vatican was closed to the public for the night, Swiss Guards were still on duty.

On October 11, the halfway point of our pilgrimage, we rose for Morning Prayer and Mass with our Franciscan hosts. An elderly Italian priest said Mass in English. One of the sisters recommended a tour of the Excavations beneath the Vatican in lieu of the catacombs we'd intended to see. She wrote "Ufficio Scavi" on a piece of paper, and instructed us to give it to the Swiss Guards.

When we presented Sister's paper to the Guards, they directed us to the *ufficio*, where we were put on the list for an afternoon tour. Through pouring rain, we then hurried into St. Peter's Basilica. It was awesome! Huge and magnificent, it can hold 80,000 people. Mass was being celebrated at one of the side altars, but it was relatively quiet that morning as we wandered about in the sanctified space.

In the afternoon, a small group of us was welcomed by a second-year seminarian from Seattle, Washington, who was studying in Rome. The young man took us down into the excavation area beneath the basilica. We were shown several ancient tombs, including St. Peter's, where we learned that the bones in his tomb aren't Peter's! We stared in stunned disappointment. But our seminarian was saving the best for last. The bones believed to be Peter's were eventually found hidden in a crypt built into the wall of his tomb. That's why the crypt marker in the upper basilica is off centre. It was constructed that way by early Christians to align with the secret crypt, and not the tomb itself. I found myself crying, so moved was I by this account of our faith's beginnings.

The next morning, as we explored the city, we were joined by a middle-aged priest who personally escorted us past Swiss Guards and in and out of official buildings. He seemed to command respect wherever he went. Before bidding farewell to our accommodating guide, Jim asked him to pose for a photo with Kevin, and to give Kevin a blessing. He obliged, and when we asked for his name and address, he told us that he was Bishop Paul Karatas of Istanbul, Turkey. He added that life had become much harder for Christians under the new Muslim government in Turkey. I bless that dear, unassuming man for his kindness to three total strangers who were shown Jesus in the person of one of the Church's humble shepherds.

Jim, Kevin and I then went to the Vatican Museum to admire tapestries, statues, paintings, mosaics, and sacred vessels. We moved slowly through the Sistine Chapel, crammed with Saturday crowds, all eyes focused upward on Michelangelo's wonderful ceiling. That night Kevin told us that if he were healed, he wished to become a priest. He didn't want to study in Rome, he said, because he would need assistance for a while.

After a return train ride from Rome, we drove through the hills and badlands to Montepulciano, a medieval walled town with steeply winding streets. From there, we did a day trip to lovely Siena with its large centre *campo*, beautiful cathedral, the Duoma, and Catherine of Siena's sanctuary. On the way back to Montepulciano, we marvelled at the unique scenery and saw several hilltops occupied by remarkable walled villages. Jim and Kevin went out that night to watch a movie being filmed outside the cathedral. It was a dramatic scene with 60 actors and someone being torched. Although they couldn't understand the Italian dialogue, Kevin found it fascinating to see a film production first hand.

In mid-afternoon of the following day, we approached Assisi. How breathtaking it was to see it sparkling on the hillside, more exotic even than the pictures in my imagination! Within these ancient walls, Francesco Giovanni Bernadone was born into the merchant class in 1182. At age 20, he was imprisoned during a battle engagement, but three years later went off to war again. A dream instructed him to return to Assisi, and later, the voice of Jesus spoke to him from the crucifix in the San Damiano chapel. By 1209, Francis and a few men were living in the valley below Assisi at the Portiuncula, a chapel previously owned by Benedictines. The brothers lived in huts encircling the little church, begging for food, preaching in the surrounding towns, and caring for lepers. Francis was indeed radical, but he was radical within the Church he loved.

In 1212, Clare of Assisi, a member of the nobility, joined Francis. She readily adopted Francis' love of poverty and gospel living. Hers was a call to mysticism and community. She became a confidante of Francis and his friars, had a gift for healing, and brought rich insights to the Franciscan movement. Francis gave Clare and her sisters San Damiano as their chapel and convent. Both Francis and Clare developed a Rule of Life for their Orders.

Today there are three branches of friars in the Franciscan First Order. Clare's followers are known as the Franciscan Second Order, or Poor Clares. From the earliest days of Franciscanism, men and women living in their own homes also began to follow the Franciscan way of life. This Third Order consists today of three branches: lay people called Secular Franciscans, religious known as Third Order Regular, and about 470 additional Franciscan religious congregations.

When we arrived in Assisi, we went first to St. Anthony's Guest House, where three Franciscan Sisters of the Atonement, Margaret, Maria, and Sue from Vancouver, welcomed us and showed us around. We then set out for an initiation tour of Assisi. How beautiful it is! We visited the nearby Basilica of St. Clare, prayed at her tomb and before the San Damiano crucifix that spoke to St. Francis. And yes, we browsed through the town's quaint little shops.

We spent Wednesday at the Basilica of St. Francis, basking in the Franciscan spirituality captured so movingly in Cimabue's paintings and Giotto's frescoes of the life of Francis. We visited Francis' crypt, and viewed his tattered robe. In the evening we walked the ancient streets, imagining the young Clare hurrying home on these same stones. We envisioned Francis preaching and begging in the village square.

The world would be shocked two years later when, in 1998, a major earthquake would devastate the historical basilicas, art masterpieces, quaint stone buildings, and much of Assisi. Major restoration and renovation projects are still transforming the famous city back to its medieval splendour.

After Thursday Morning Prayer, we walked to San Damiano, convent of Clare and her sisters, and site of the crucifix that spoke to the young Francis. The church was closed for restoration, but we were able to visit St. Clare's choir, garden, chapel and dormitory. It is a place of serenity and simple beauty. Pilgrims walk through the rooms and gardens with quiet reverence.

As we paused on our 1.5-kilometre walk back to Assisi, Kevin began to type that St. Clare had spoken to him in the dormitory. She told him he would have to be patient and work hard in order to be normal, he typed. She told him that he would be much better soon, that Jesus loved him, and that he would be whole in heaven where all his friends and family would be with him.

We continued silently down the road, absorbing this strange information. When we again stopped for a rest, I somewhat skeptically asked Kevin what St. Clare's voice was like. He typed, "I did not hear her voice, but I felt her in my senses."

"In your mind?" I asked.

And he said, "Not as much in my mind as in my senses. I could smell her and she smelled fresh like soap and water, and I could feel her sweetness and gentleness, and I wanted to be in her arms, clasped to her self. And as far as I can tell, Jesus was also there, and I could feel his gentleness and sadness for the world, and he wants me to pray for all people as if I were in a cloister because I am in a cloister."

The road between San Damiano and Assisi curves gently among olive groves. The three of us continued wordlessly along this road, bonded by our touch with eternity. Kevin had introduced us to the mystic Clare, and we believed. God was very near. I pondered Clare's words: be patient, work hard, much better soon. I contemplated Kevin's words for Jesus: gentleness, sadness, pray. I understood that we were being asked to endure, to join our lives with the suffering Christ, and to do so with hope.

Kevin remained subdued all day, even through an enjoyable dinner at the convent. Later he confirmed that he was struggling to come to terms with the fact that Clare had not promised him a quick and total cure. I reminded him that Jesus was always with him – and some day he would be well.

On Friday we reluctantly left the guest house. In the valley below Assisi, we stopped at the massive Cathedral of Santa Maria d'Angeli which had been built to protect the Portiuncula. Within its walls, the little chapel, birthplace of Franciscanism, is dwarfed and reverenced by the larger building. It so happened that, on the day of our visit, a family was celebrating an anniversary Mass within the Portiuncula. Several observers stood outside Francis' tiny chapel, and Jim, Kevin and some others were able to receive communion there. In Santa Maria's gift shop, we bought a rosary requested by a Franciscan friend and obtained a poster showing the Portiuncula surrounded by tiny huts as in Francis' time.

From there, we travelled along the Italian Riviera and through the wee kingdom of Monaco. On a warm, sunny morning complete with blue skies and a matching Mediterranean Sea, we returned to France, followed hilly, walled roads, and drove through beach towns on the Côte d'Azur. Past Aix-en-Provence, we enjoyed lunch overlooking the sea, and reached Avignon at dusk. We were awed by Avignon, and the fairy-tale walls surrounding this magnificent city of fourteenth-century popes.

Once we had crossed into Spain, thick smog forced us back from Barcelona, and we ended up in Cardova. Impulsively, we decided to stay at a wonderful mountaintop castle the government operates as a hotel. In the evening, we stood at our window, high up in the castle wall. Numerous bats swooped silently by the open window, which was protected only by a grate covering the bottom quarter. Kevin expressed alarm about the window, and told us he was angry that we had taken him to such frightening places as Venice and this castle. Then he admitted that he was really feeling anxious about Lourdes. He was so hoping for the miracle of speech.

I awoke in the middle of the night and stood again at the castle window. The sky glittered with stars. Streetlights in the village below and winding up the castle road were shrouded in soft fog. It was spellbinding: traces of human presence amidst the timelessness and immensity of Creation.

The following day, we set off through the Apennines. Some of the roads through Spain's mountains were narrow and scary. Kevin said the ride was "terrible," and that we "should have known better than to come this way." He ate little all day, and seemed unwell when we arrived at our hotel near the grotto at Lourdes. Nonetheless, he was eager to go out, and was delighted with the candle-lit rosary held below the Basilica. When we returned to our hotel, he was feverish, so I gave him medication and put him to bed.

In the morning, he seemed slightly better, and insisted on going to the baths. Jim and Kevin went in together, and Kevin came out smiling. He typed, "I am happy and hopeful that I will lead a useful life and serve Jesus as Mary wishes. I may still be autistic but I will be able to lead a useful life. I want to tell Bishop Sherlock that I am a different man. Possibly I am healed of my addiction to butts. Most of all, I feel that my spirit is healed and I have dignity."

Kevin was very feverish and vomiting during the night. In the morning, though, he wished to go to the shrine again and "touch the rock." At the shrine, he walked about with his hands in prayer position. Back at the hotel, he typed that he felt he had been in the "holy presence of Mary and Jesus. As far as I can tell, I am to live a life imitating the suffering of Christ and praying for the world. I am to be an example of peace and hopefulness for others."

## Spiritual journey

Despite my concern for Kevin's health, I returned from the European pilgrimage determined and optimistic about his future. A person with Kevin's courage, compassion and desire to have a meaningful life deserves the same opportunities as others. I felt that I was being called to be less complacent and more persistent in helping him follow his dreams.

The process of pilgrimage activates our courage to continue to seek healing from God and God's human healers. "There are seldom magical solutions – instant healings in our lives," says Bodo, "but there is always the operation of grace, that mysterious gift of God's divine life in us drawing us closer to union with God."[2]

Throughout our lifetimes, we travel relentlessly eastward towards the Rising Sun, towards the Creator God who loved us into being. We travel multi-dimensionally with seen and unseen presences. We travel with our memories of the past, and with our dreams for the future. We plod along even when we lose sight of the light or forget that we are pilgrims. The paths we take include bumps, dips, stretches of shadow, and places of breathtaking beauty. There can be seemingly unbearable darkness, and glimpses of tantalizing light.

> Our carefree, joyous times are the mountaintops
> where everything is beautiful and refreshing.
> Periods of sorrow, depression and trouble
> are the valleys.
> Mountaintops are restful and exhilarating
> and we should treasure our times there.
> In valleys, growth takes place
> in the rain and the fertile soil.
> We must learn to accept, and even be grateful,
> for both.[3]

We learn to accept and appreciate the exhilaration felt on mountaintops as well as the growing pains of valleys. We learn, too, that pilgrimage is a community experience. Even hermit nuns and monks emerge periodically from their contemplative silence to worship, work and break bread with others. Followers of Catherine Doherty, trained by her in eastern spirituality, "came to embrace the full vocation of the Russian *poustinik* of three days in and four days out."[4]

Early in our European pilgrimage, we realized we had far too much luggage. We had arrived in Paris wearing our multi-pocketed tourist vests, while carrying one backpack plus one large, heavy bag each. All of this had to be toted as we climbed aboard bus and subway, or walked Parisian streets. As soon as we acquired the Renault, we did a complete re-pack.

The backpacks became carriers of food, water, and other travel necessities. Toiletries and clothing for the three of us were packed into *one* suitcase. Since public laundromats are scarce in Europe, clothing is best washed nightly by hand. Easy wash, fast dry is the rule of thumb when choosing travel clothes. Our two remaining suitcases were stowed in the trunk of the Renault for the remainder of the trip, redundant and unused.

The lessons of pilgrimage translate well when applied to daily life. The more we have, the more we have to carry. The simpler our lives, the more we enjoy what's really important. Most lessons are best learned through direct experience. Just as we were jolted by the stark reality of Dachau, more often than not it takes a sobering close-to-the-heart experience to remind us that we are not in control of destiny. And the most important lesson is trust.

Trust in God brings its own kind of peace. It quiets restlessness and calms anxiety. Throughout this pilgrimage, Kevin was hoping for a miracle at Lourdes. So whenever we visited a church – which was often, due to the abundance and splendour of European churches – we prayed for Kevin's miracle. I reminded him, as I reminded myself, that the only important miracle is entry into heaven.

The external journey of pilgrimage is to the place of healing. The inner journey is a "pilgrimage into the soul, where God dwells, the place in which we receive healing and become channels of healing for each other. We were bringing with us the very God we were travelling to find."[5] But we had to search for God and travel towards God in order to discover the source of our quest.

While we are growing more intimate in our relationship with God, our fear of the unknown lessens. We accept loss and suffering as part of the weave. We believe that the complete tapestry is in the hands of God, and that all will be well. All *is* well.

Thomas Merton reminds us that we need not carry our burdens alone. Once our lives become God-centred, we lose our tragic, self-important seriousness and take only God seriously. To take God seriously "is to find joy and spontaneity in everything, for everything is gift and grace." When we become aware of the cosmic dance, and "move in time with the Dancer," says Merton, "our life attains its true dimension. It is at once more serious and less serious than the life of one who does not sense this inner cosmic dynamism."[6]

"Life can be complicated and difficult and sometimes hard to understand," says Kevin, "but when we turn things over to God, everything becomes easy and clear and beautiful. I will continue to seek miracles because miracles are all around us. God is close by, and my grandparents are watching over me."

And so our story ends, but not the journey. We continue to read the maps and follow the roads that lead to the next destination. We travel in hope because God is love. We travel in peace because, as a pilgrim community, we are never alone.

# As Far As I Can Tell

As far as I can tell, I have always been a Franciscan at heart. Even before I learned that Francis is the patron of ecology, I was fascinated by the saint who loved the earth and all its creatures. By the time I joined the Secular Franciscan Order, I was seeking a deeper relationship with God and pursuing the joy of Francis. Only gradually would I come to appreciate that Francis' *perfect joy* came from his acceptance of suffering.

As you will have noticed, Kevin regularly uses the phrase "as far as I can tell" in conversation. He explains that he does this so he is "not dictating [his] opinions." Such is his gentle nature. He certainly has opinions, but because of his vulnerability, he has never been in a position of power. Like all the voiceless ones of the earth, others have dictated to him. Francis, too, had opinions: opinions that he generously shared, but never dictated.

As far as I can tell, it is in my nature to dictate and control, as it is to be proud, possessive and stubborn. It has taken me years to begin to understand the joy of Francis. It has taken me years to realize that whenever I *think* I have the joy or the simplicity or the humility of Jesus and Francis, then I truly don't.

In an outpouring of joyful praise during the last year of his life, Francis of Assisi created his final song, *The Canticle of Brother Sun*. It brilliantly encapsulates Franciscan spirituality, reconciliation with all of creation, and the male–female dimensions of the soul.

*Most High, all-powerful, good Lord,*
*Yours are the praises, the glory, the honour, and all blessing.*
*To You alone, do they belong,*
*and no one is worthy to mention Your name.*

As far as I can tell, God likes to be talked to honestly, as we would talk to a friend. I expect that Francis, in his lifetime, sometimes cried out to God in doubt and despair, as I have. Like the Psalmist, he sometimes shouted in anger. Franciscan spirituality tells us to pray to God from our experience of the moment. When Francis sang to *the most-high, all-powerful, good Lord*, he was at that moment rejoicing in the conviction that God had been faithful to him through thick and thin, just as Francis had remained faithful to God.

*Praised be You, my Lord, with all Your creatures,*
*especially Sir Brother Sun,*
*Who is the day and through whom You give us light.*
*And he is beautiful and radiant with great splendour;*
*and bears a likeness of You, Most High One.*

As far as I can tell, each day would be enhanced through seeing in Brother Sun the Son *who is the day...gives us light...is beautiful and radiant...and bears a likeness of You, Most High One.* The image of the mirror was central to Clare of Assisi's spirituality. Clare saw Francis as the mirror of Christ. In the poor Christ, she saw the mirror we are to contemplate. Franciscan spirituality is the essence of Christian spirituality because it embraces the simplicity, humility and compassion of Jesus. Were I to look into the mirror that is Christ-in-the-poor and see myself, I could become a mirror to the world.

*Praised be You, my Lord, through Sister Moon and the stars,*
*in heaven You formed them clear and precious and beautiful.*

As far as I can tell, many would consider Francis a fool and Clare a misguided recluse. But Francis, dreamer and visionary, and Clare, mystic and healer, were as *clear, precious and beautiful* in the sight of God as they perceived *Sister Moon and the stars* to be. When we detach our hearts from property, possessions and power, we adopt a spiritual poverty that the world ridicules. But when the map of our inner vision is lit by the light of Christ, the journey's safety is assured.

*Praised be You, my Lord, through Brother Wind,*
*and through the air, cloudy and serene, and every kind of weather*
*through which You give sustenance to Your creatures.*

As far as I can tell, it took me a while to know with certainty that limitations and imperfections are as beautiful and awesome as *every kind of weather* borne by *Brother Wind*. Furthermore, limitations and imperfections are as necessary as *every kind of weather*. Just as each snowflake is unique and pottery is valued for its imperfections, so are we individually called by name and cherished by the Creator. Franciscan spirituality can be fully lived by people with different lifestyles, different personalities and different capabilities.

*Praised be You, my Lord, through Sister Water,*
*which is very useful and humble and precious and chaste.*

As far as I can tell, Francis attributed to water that which was beautiful in him. Francis would have readily recognized these attributes in Christ, but not in himself. Like Sister Water, Francis was *very useful and humble and precious and chaste*. Through living the gospel of Jesus Christ, both Francis and Clare embraced community lifestyles. After all, to be human is to need to live in relationship with others. Thus, the spirituality of Francis draws us in the dark times of our lives. In emulating Clare and Francis, we become comfortable with our place in life.

*Praised be You, my Lord, through Brother Fire,*
*through whom You light the night*
*and he is beautiful and playful and robust and strong.*

As far as I can tell, Francis and Clare would not be intimidated by the state of the world today. After all, there was much about the twelfth century that, like the 21st century, was bleak, violent and terrifying. The Church had major problems, too. The saints of Assisi simply approached each difficulty as something to be changed. Fight fire with fire! Thus encouraged, we can thank God that we're alive now to bring peace and joy ... to fight evil ... to care for creation. For me, St. Francis Advocates, through their ministry with the vulnerable, light the night, as does Brother Fire. For the disabled and their families, it is also *beautiful and playful and robust and strong*.

*Praised be You, my Lord, through our Sister Mother Earth,*
*who sustains and governs us,*
*and who produces varied fruits with coloured flowers and herbs.*

As far as I can tell, our Sister Mother Earth needs a big apology. The same abuse and negligence we heap upon our bodies, we bestow on our beautiful planet. In fact, the time for apology is past, and we must hasten to search for healing for us all. Kevin struggles with his addictions and obsessions. We focus on him because of his dependence on us, but we all have addictions and obsessions. I turn to Francis for help and see that he, finding God in creation, praised God through all creatures.

Therefore I take heart and will praise God in my care of the earth: its flora, fauna and peoples.

*Praised be You, my Lord, through those who give pardon for Your love*
*and bear infirmity and tribulation.*
*Blessed are those who endure in peace*
*for by You, Most High, they shall be crowned.*

As far as I can tell, no one is exempt from infirmity and tribulation. This is a blessing, because we obtain Franciscan peace and perfect joy through suffering. Francis was able to draw on the experiences of his life – imprisonment, illness, depression, deprivation, approach of death, rejection, ridicule. In embracing suffering, he received peace and a deeper union with God.

As far as I can tell, when we surrender our suffering to God, we feel peace and joy sprouting in the mulch of our darkness. Entering the silence in the depths of our souls, we come face to face with our failures, limitations, sinfulness, loneliness, rejection and fears. It is then we feel the stirrings of peace and joy: knowing we have God's love.

The final verses of the Canticle were composed by Francis at the Portiuncula as he was dying.

*Praised be You, my Lord, through our Sister Bodily Death,*
*from whom no living man can escape.*
*Woe to those who die in mortal sin.*
*Blessed are those whom death will find in Your most holy will,*
*for the second death shall do them no harm.*

As far as I can tell, praising God through Sister Bodily Death grew naturally from Francis' acceptance of suffering and his absorption in the life of Jesus. He guided Clare and her sisters towards this peace by telling them to live always in truth, so as to die in obedience to the divine will, which wishes only good for all. Do not look at the life outside, said Francis, for that of the Spirit is better.

As far as I can tell, Kevin does not seem afraid of dying. In fact, he has said that he wants to die when I die. He has a greater fear of being left on the earth without parents. But then, heaven for Kevin means being whole and safe with God.

*Praise and bless my Lord and give Him thanks*
*and serve Him with great humility.*

As far as I can tell, personal suffering in ourselves or shared with others transforms our lives to ones of prayer, gospel living and perfect joy. Being the parent of a vulnerable child has led me on a long and multi-dimensional quest. Franciscan spirituality has shown me the paradox of joy in suffering. Francis understood that the difference between fleeting bursts of happiness and perfect joy is simply the willingness to bear hardship for Christ.

# Notes

**1   Communication**

[1]   Temple Grandin, "Needs of High Functioning Teenagers and Adults with Autism: Tips from a Recovered Autistic" in *Focus on Autistic Behavior*, Richard Simpson, ed. Vol. 5, No. 1, April 1990, 7.

[2]   M.-Marsel Mesulam, "Neural Substrates of Behavior: The Effects of Focal Brain Lesions upon Mental State" in *The Harvard Guide to Psychiatry, Third Edition*. Armand M. Nicholi, Jr., M.D., ed. (Cambridge: The Belnap Press of Harvard University Press, 1999), 112.

[3]   Douglas Biklen, "Communication Unbound: Autism and Praxis" in *Harvard Educational Review*, Vol. 60, No. 3, August 1990, 297.

[4]   But FC is still not without its critics or its difficulties. To begin with, how does one explain that most of the users had been considered intellectually subnormal prior to their astonishing communications?

Author Charles Hart, who has both a brother and a son with autism, believes that there are several subtypes of autism. Children who progress normally through speech development until shortly before their second birthdays, like David Eastham and our Kevin, may be a subtype. Hart says of facilitated communication,

It seems that some children have a progressive form of apraxia that destroys verbal communication. Perhaps they have a subtype that has no intellectual limits, merely neuromotor interference with speech. They may have the intellectual capacity to think, emote, and communicate, but can't perform the physical movements...necessary to speak. (Charles A. Hart, *A Parents Guide to Autism* [New York: Pocket Books, 1993], 178.)

The Ontario Consultants on Religious Tolerance, an agency that promotes religious tolerance and presents all sides on various controversial issues, also believes that only those with higher intelligence can use FC effectively. These, it feels, should move on to independent typing as soon as possible. "Autism is a generic label applied to persons who exhibit a group of symptoms," reports an article by B.A. Robinson on the Tolerance website. "The vast majority are diagnosed correctly as having a severe intellectual deficit. For them, FC is useless as anything other than a game. A small minority are of near normal (or even superior) intelligence but are unable to speak because of neuromotor impairment. Some of the latter can proceed to independent typing, by using FC as a temporary crutch." (B.A. Robinson, "What Is Facilitated Communication [FC & FCT]?", Ontario

Consultants on Religious Tolerance, 2001, 13.)

Another criticism concerns the fact that many of these users have not been taught to read. How, then, can they converse so wisely? Is it not more likely that the facilitator, consciously or otherwise, is influencing the communication?

Biklen writes,

Crossley's students and their parents typically report that the students had had incidental exposure to language through television, magazines, and books, or with labels on foods and other items. Some were reported to have been in formal reading programs as part of early intervention and developmental training efforts. Yet until Crossley elicited typing from them, the assumption for all of them was that they had not learned to read (Biklen, 297).

To that I would add that most of these individuals have sat in classrooms for years, silently observing and absorbing knowledge that they were unable to acknowledge either verbally or in writing.

Then there is the criticism that accusations of sexual abuse, arising during facilitated communication sessions, have disrupted some families. This is indeed tragic. On the other hand, it is well known that a higher percentage of disabled persons are sexually abused than in the general population. The only opportunity that many would have to make this injustice and their terrible suffering known would be through a facilitator.

A fourth criticism is that users usually do not perform well in quantitative, objective testing. They have trouble dealing with an unfamiliar environment, strange equipment such as blindfolds and earphones, and the presence of observers.

Promoters of FC prefer studies that have the qualitative methodologies used by anthropologists and educators. They like to avoid confrontational study techniques that might undermine the user's self-confidence. Biklen says that many users require additional time to answer questions, and often need two or three tries. Users also need to be reminded to focus on the keyboard and not to gaze about.

And what of the criticism that only a few benefit from facilitated communication? I see this as a challenge rather than a criticism. How do we know for certain who can benefit? Successful users of FC were often seen as intellectually deficient prior to having the opportunity to communicate. Furthermore, should any human being, regardless of ability, be deprived of their right to be heard?

Critics also protest the pressure to accept FC uncritically. They say that because typical attempts to communicate with people with autism are often futile, and conventional treatments and techniques work poorly, if at all, parents and caregivers are desperate for a breakthrough. Facilitators themselves may feel under intense pressure to make FC work. "If they are unsuccessful at showing results, they may feel a loss of self-esteem, and a loss of status among their coworkers. Ultimately, they may fear a loss of employment. These factors contribute to an intense desire to produce results. This might induce some facilitators to guide the hand of the user – perhaps without realizing it," says Robinson (Robinson, 4-5).

To the contrary, I believe there should be *more* pressure to try facilitated communication, not less. Of course parents and caregivers are desperate for a communication breakthrough! Of course facilitators want FC to work!

5    Jean Vanier, *Drawn into the Mystery of Jesus Through the Gospel of John* (Ottawa: Novalis, 2004), 106.

6    Robinson, 2.

7    Elizabeth Bloomfield, personal letter to author, October 2, 2003.

8    M. Scott Peck, *The Different Drum: Community Making and Peace* (New York: Touchstone, 1989), 257.

9    Kathleen Norris, "From Dakota: A Spiritual Geography" in *Pilgrim Souls: A Collection of Spiritual Autobiographies*, Amy Mandelker & Elizabeth Powers, eds. (New York: Touchstone, 1999), 143.

## 2    Community

1    John P. Radford & Deborah C. Park, "Historical Overview of Developmental Disabilities in Ontario" in *Developmental Disabilities in Ontario*, Ivan Brown and Maire Percy, eds. (Toronto: Front Porch Publishing, 1999), 5.

2    Harold Cardinal, *The Unjust Society* (Vancouver: Douglas & McIntyre, 1985), 46.

3    Radford & Park, 1.

4    Radford & Park, 1.

5    Radford & Park, 1.

6    Radford & Park, 9.

7    M. Scott Peck, *The Different Drum: Community Making and Peace* (New York: Touchstone, 1989), 60.

8    Peck, 61.

9    Rabbi Hayim Halevy Donin, *To Pray as a Jew: A Guide to the Prayer Book and the Synagogue Service* (New York: Basic Books, 1980), 3.

10    Richard Rohr, *Simplicity: The Freedom of Letting Go* (New York: Crossroad, 2003), 182.

11    Ingrid J. Peterson, O.S.F., *Clare of Assisi: A Biographical Study* (Quincy, IL: Franciscan Press, 1993), 177.

12    "The Rule of Saint Clare" in *Francis and Clare: The Complete Works* (New York: Paulist

Press, 1982), 216.

[13] *The Rule of the Secular Franciscan Order*, article iv.

[14] Murray Bodo, *The Place We Call Home: Spiritual Pilgrimage as a Path to God* (Brewster, MA: Paraclete Press, 2004), 7.

### 3  Adjusting

[1] Catherine M. Lee and Ian H. Gotlib. "Mental Illness and the Family" in *Handbook of Developmental Family Psychology and Psychopathology*, Luciano L'Abate, ed. (New York: John Wiley & Sons Inc., 1994), 248.

[2] Lee and Gotlib, 248.

[3] Janice Mawhinney, "MD Delves into Autistic Minds," *The Toronto Star* (Tuesday, January 6, 1998), B3.

[4] Lee and Gotlib, 248.

[5] Jean Vanier, *Our Journey Home* (Ottawa: Novalis, 1997), 35.

[6] Richard Rohr, *Simplicity: The Freedom of Letting Go* (New York: Crossroad, 2003), 29.

[7] Richard Leonard SJ, *Beloved Daughters: 100 Years of Papal Teaching on Women* (Toronto: Novalis, 1995), 108–109.

[8] Leonard, 109–110.

[9] Rohr, 31.

[10] Marie-Louise Ternier-Gommers, *Finding the Treasure Within: A Woman's Journey into Preaching* (Ottawa: Novalis, 2002), 237.

[11] Ron Rolheiser, "A Healthy Church Includes Many Voices," *The Catholic Register* (Week of January 23, 2005), 19.

[12] Rohr, 60.

### 4  Addiction

[1] Allen Frances, M.D. and Michael B. First, M.D, *Your Mental Health: A Layman's Guide to the Psychiatrist's Bible* (New York: Scribner, 1998), 138.

[2] Michael Swan, "Reaching out to the Addicted," *The Catholic Register* (Week of October 12, 2003), 10.

[3] Gabrielle Roy, *Where Nests the Water Hen* (Toronto: McClelland & Stewart, 1989), 30.

[4] Jean Vanier, *An Ark for the Poor: The Story of L'Arche* (Ottawa: Novalis, 1995), 119.

[5] The founding board of directors of St. Francis Advocates consisted of nine

dedicated friends. Reta Mitro, office clerk and test-car driver for Imperial Oil Ltd., became president, and I, vice-president. Mary Mitro, part owner and office manager of Up-Rite Door Ltd., was the very hard-working secretary-treasurer. Deborah Austin, barrister with the firm of Wyrzykowski, Higgins and Austin, contributed invaluable legal counsel. Ronald Savage, teaching master at Lambton College, was property chairman, and Charles Oxley, marketing manager of emulsion rubber for Polysar Ltd., was the board's financial adviser.

The three other founding board directors were Bro. Anthony VandenHeuvel, Brother of St. Louis and family life education director for the Lambton County Separate School Board; Hildy Wyrzykowski, a talented amateur photographer; and Sr. Mary Margaret Howard, Sister of St. Joseph and pastoral assistant at St. Joseph's parish, Sarnia, Ontario.

6   By late 1987, the Board of Directors had seen some changes. Reta, Mary and I retained our offices, as did directors Ron Savage and Debbie Austin. New to St. Francis Advocates were directors Keith Sharpe, teacher at Gregory Hogan school, Sarnia; my brother, Thomas Pearson, process operator, Dow Chemical, Sarnia; William Morkin, principal, Father Gerald LaBelle school, Corunna; and Janice Brown, teacher, St. Peter Canisius school, Watford. Bramwell Gregson was hired as our consultant.

7   Jean Vanier, *Man and Woman He Made Them* (London, UK: Darton, Longman and Todd, 1985), 156.

8   Frances, 132.

9   Frances, 139.

10  Jane E. Brody, "Knowing When to Stop," *National Post* (Thursday, October 9, 2003), A19.

11  Roy Barkley, *Catholic Ministry to the Addicted* (Huntington, IN: Our Sunday Visitor Publishing Division, 1992), 46.

12  Barkley, 100.

13  Barkley, 119.

14  Barkley, 73.

### 5   Resources

1   Geneva Centre for Autism (www.autism.net/index.php) provides information and service to persons with autism and their families.

2   Author's notes, August 1976.

3   Several of these resources include the following:

- Autism Society Canada (www.autisimsocietycanada.ca) publishes an online newsletter and lists links to other important Autism Spectrum Disorders information.

- Autism Society Ontario (www.autismsociety.on.ca) publishes a newsletter and provides information and services to its members. (1179A King Street West, Suite 004, Toronto, ON, Canada M6K 3C5; Tel: 1-800-472-7789).

- Autism Society of America (ASA) publishes a newsletter and provides information and services to its members. (7910 Woodmont Avenue, Suite 300, Bethesda, MD, USA 20814-3067; Tel: 1-800-328-8476 or 1-301-657-0881).

- Charles A. Hart, *A Parent's Guide to Autism*. (New York: Pocket Books, 1993). Contains excellent resource listings. The author has both a brother and a son with autism.

- *Autism Research Review International*, Bernard Rimland, ed. Quarterly publication of Autism Research International (4182 Adams Avenue, San Diego, CA, USA 92116). This informative newsletter reviews research trends. Produced by psychologist Bernard Rimland, father of a son with autism.

- Autism Spectrum Disorders – Canadian American Research Consortium (Autism Research Program, c/o Ongwanada Resource Centre, 191 Portsmouth Avenue, Kingston, ON Canada K7M 8A6; Tel: 1-866-273-2272). Consider participating in a research program. The Autism Spectrum Disorders – Canadian American Research Consortium is a multi-disciplinary team composed of more than 60 researchers, clinicians and parents dedicated to unravelling the mystery of autism.

[4] Sister Frances Teresa osc, *This Living Mirror: Reflections on Clare of Assisi* (Maryknoll, NY: Orbis, 1995), 72.

## 6   Relationships

[1] In 1988, Gerry Mak of Lambton Engineering was our architect, and Ray Wyrzykowski was our lawyer. At the SFA annual meeting on October 26, 1988, the following slate of officers was elected: Gloria Pearson-Vasey, president; Reta Mitro, past president; Mary Mitro, vice-president; Bill Morkin, secretary; and Tom Kelly, treasurer. New directors in 1989 were William Hemstreet and Joseph Palko. Diane Kemsley provided secretarial services, and John Beer was accounting consultant.

[2] Temple Grandin, "Needs of High Functioning Teenagers and Adults with Autism: Tips from a Recovered Autistic" in *Focus on Autistic Behavior*, Richard Simpson, ed. Vol. 5, No. 1, April 1990, 1.

[3] Thomas and Donna Finn, *Intimate Bedfellows: Love, Sex, and the Catholic Church* (Boston: Pauline Books & Media, 1993), 19.

[4] Jean Vanier, *Man and Woman He Made Them* (London, UK: Darton, Longman and Todd, 1985), 156.

[5] Grandin, 7.

6   Armand M. Nicholi, Jr., "The Adolescent" in *The Harvard Guide to Psychiatry, Third Edition*, Armand M. Nicholi, Jr., M.D., ed. (Cambridge: The Belnap Press of Harvard University Press, 1999), 621–622.

7   Mary Alban Bouchard, *Overcoming Loneliness Together: A Christian Approach* (Ottawa: Novalis, 1991), 254.

8   Vanier, 61.

9   On February 27, 2003, I attended a workshop on sexuality and Christian commitment in London, Ontario, entitled "The Pervasive Nature of Sexuality." The presenter was Raymond F. Dlugos, OSA, Ph.D., from the Southdown Institute, Guelph.

10  Richard Rohr, *Simplicity: The Freedom of Letting Go* (New York: Crossroad, 2003), 154.

11  Henri J.M. Nouwen, *The Road to Daybreak: A Spiritual Journey* (New York: Image Books, 1988), 169.

12  Murray Bodo, *The Way of St. Francis: The Challenge of Franciscan Spirituality for Everyone* (Cincinnati, OH: St. Anthony Messenger Press, 1995), 58.

13  Sister Frances Teresa osc, *This Living Mirror: Reflections on Clare of Assisi* (Maryknoll, NY: Orbis, 1995), 94.

## 7  Hope and Dreams

1   Temple Grandin, "Teaching Tips from a Recovered Autistic" in *Focus on Autistic Behavior*, Richard Simpson, ed. Vol. 3, No, 1, April 1988, 6.

2   Sister Frances Teresa osc, *This Living Mirror: Reflections on Clare of Assisi* (New York: Maryknoll, NY: Orbis, 1995), 94.

3   Viktor E. Frankl, "From Experiences in a Concentration Camp" in *Pilgrim Souls: A Collection of Spiritual Autobiographies*, Amy Mandelker and Elizabeth Powers, eds. (Chicago: Franciscan Herald Press, 1983), 493.

4   "Mirror of Perfection" in *St. Francis of Assisi Omnibus of Sources*, Marion A. Habig, ed. (Chicago: Franciscan Herald Press, 1983), 1230.

5   V.C. Keating, *The Fire Stone* (Victoria, BC: Trafford, 2004), 182.

6   Patti Normile, *Following Francis of Assisi: A Spirituality for Daily Living* (Cincinnati, OH: St. Anthony Messenger Press, 1996), 109.

7   Charles Theisler, *Migraine: Winning the Fight Of Your Life* (Lancaster, PA: Starburst Publishers, 1995), 108–109.

8   *The Rule of the Secular Franciscan Order*, article viii.

9   *The Rule of the Secular Franciscan Order*, article iv.

## 8  Limitations

1. Murray Bodo, *The Way of St. Francis: The Challenge of Franciscan Spirituality for Everyone* (Cincinnati, OH: St. Anthony Messenger Press, 1995), 87.
2. William R. Hugo, OFM Cap. *Studying the Life of Francis of Assisi: A Beginner's Workbook* (Quincy, IL: Franciscan Press, 1996), 15–16.
3. Temple Grandin, "Needs of High Functioning Teenagers and Adults with Autism: Tips from a Recovered Autistic" in *Focus on Autistic Behavior*, Richard Simpson, ed. Vol. 5, No. 1, April 1990, 12.
4. Catherine R. Gugerty, S.S.N.D. "From Guilt to Gratitude: Spiritual Ministry with Persons Who Are Poor and Homeless" in *Handbook of Spirituality for Ministers*, Robert J. Wicks, ed. (New York: Paulist Press, 1995), 477.
5. V.C. Keating, *Meditative Moments: A New Testament Year* (Victoria, BC: Trafford, 2004), 120.
6. *The Merck Manual of Medical Information: Home Edition*, Robert Berkow, M.D., Mark H. Beers, M.D., and Andrew J. Fletcher, eds. (Whitehouse Station, NJ: Merck Research Laboratories, 1997), 428.
7. Richard Rohr, *Simplicity: The Freedom of Letting Go* (New York: Crossroad, 2003), 147.
8. Sister Frances Teresa, osc, *This Living Mirror: Reflections on Clare of Assisi* (Maryknoll, NY: Orbis, 1995), 94.
9. The genetic connection is vague at present, but science may prove a link at some point in the future. There are a few families with two or more autistic children. If you extend the definition of autism to include Fragile X chromosomes or familial autistic behaviours, then there is evidence of a genetic connection.
10. Rohr, 147.
11. Hugo, 108.

## 9  Pioneers and Pilgrims

1. *The Birth of Special Olympics in Canada*. (contact SOC National Office at 416-927-9050 or e-mail info@specialolympics.ca).
2. Andrew Bloomfield, Newsletter, December 1, 2003.
3. Jean Vanier, *The Heart of L'Arche: A Spirituality for Every Day* (Ottawa: Novalis, 1995), 74.
4. Vanier, 74–75.
5. V.C. Keating, *Meditative Moments: A New Testament Year* (Victoria, BC: Trafford, 2004), 179.

⁶ Richard Rohr, *Simplicity: The Freedom of Letting Go* (New York: Crossroad, 2003), 60.

⁷ Sister Frances Teresa, osc, *This Living Mirror: Reflections on Clare of Assisi* (Maryknoll, NY: Orbis, 1995), 83.

⁸ Adela DiUbaldo Torchia, *Brother Fire, Sister Earth* (Ottawa: Novalis, 1993), 36.

⁹ Patti Normile, *Following Francis of Assisi: A Spirituality for Daily Living* (Cincinnati: St. Anthony Messenger Press, 1996), 67.

¹⁰ Pierre Descouvemont and Helmuth Nils Loose, *Therese and Lisieux* (Ottawa: Novalis, 2001), 226.

¹¹ Christina Spahn, "Becoming an Active Contemplative" in *Grace in Action*, Richard Rohr, ed. (New York: Crossroad, 1994), 136.

## 10 The Quest for Meaning

¹ Carolyn Gratton, *The Art of Spiritual Guidance* (New York: Crossroad, 1997), 160.

² Ron Rolheiser, "To Be Human Is to Be Pathologically Complex," *The Catholic Register* (Week of October 5, 2003), 35.

³ John R.H. Moorman, "The Franciscans" in *The Study of Spirituality*. Cheslyn Jones, Geoffrey Wainwright and Edward Yarnold, SJ, eds. (New York: Oxford University Press, 1986), 305.

⁴ Pierre Descouvemont and Helmuth Nils Loose, *Therese and Lisieux* (Ottawa: Novalis, 2001), 278.

⁵ *Francis and Clare: The Complete Works* (New York: Paulist Press, 1982), 12.

⁶ Thomas St. James O'Connor and Elizabeth Meakes, "Forgiveness and Resentment Among People with Disabilities" in *The Challenge of Forgiveness*, Augustine Meier and Peter VanKatwyk, eds. (Ottawa: Novalis, 2001), 278.

⁷ Sister Frances Teresa, osc, *This Living Mirror: Reflections on Clare of Assisi* (Maryknoll, NY: Orbis, 1995), 84.

⁸ Teresa, 83.

⁹ Moorman, 303.

## 11 Going Home

¹ Henri J.M. Nouwen, *The Wounded Healer* (New York: Image Books, 1979), 66.

² Edith Hahn Beer with Susan Dworkin, *The Nazi Officer's Wife* (New York: Rob Weisbach Books, 1999), 277.

³ U.S. Bishops. "Guidelines for Celebration of the Sacraments with Persons with

Disabilities," *Origins,* CNS Documentary Service (June 29, 1995, Vol. 25, No. 7), 107.

4   U.S. Bishops, 107.

5   U.S. Bishops, 109.

6   Richard Rohr, *Simplicity: The Freedom of Letting Go* (New York: Crossroad, 2003), 184.

7   Murray Bodo, *The Place We Call Home: Spiritual Pilgrimage as a Path to God* (Brewster, MA: Paraclete Press, 2004), 19.

8   Jean Vanier, *Our Journey Home* (Ottawa: Novalis, 1997), 129.

9   Murray Bodo, *The Way of St. Francis: The Challenge of Franciscan Spirituality for Everyone* (Cincinnati, OH: St. Anthony Messenger Press, 1995), 2.

10  Bodo, *The Way of St. Francis,* 2.

11  *Francis and Clare: The Complete Works* (New York: Paulist Press, 1982), 231.

## 12  The Advocates

1   There were greetings from the Ministry of Housing in the persons of Craig Johnson, program supervisor, and Velta Baumanis, architect. Michael Byrne, program supervisor, and Moira Elsley, program director, brought greetings from the Ministry of Community and Social Services.

2   At the annual meeting in October 1990, the following board executive was elected: Tom Pearson, president; Gloria Pearson-Vasey, past president; Janice Brown, vice-president; Catherine Lynch, secretary; and Patricia Sloan, treasurer. Directors were Father Frank White, Dr. Jack Lynch, Patricia Sloan, and Patricia Hodgetts. Dr. Stephen Hodgetts was medical consultant and John Beer was accounting consultant.

3   Murray Bodo, *The Way of St. Francis: The Challenge of Franciscan Spirituality for Everyone* (Cincinnati, OH: St. Anthony Messenger Press, 1995), 65.

4   Bodo, 65.

5   Mary Elizabeth Ingham, C.S.J. "John Duns Scotus: An Integrated Vision" in *The History of Franciscan Theology,* Kenan B. Osborne, O.F.M., ed. (St. Bonaventure, NY: The Franciscan Institute Press, 1994), 186–187.

6   Catherine de Hueck Doherty, *Poustinia* (Combermere, ON: Madonna House Publications, 1993), 53.

7   Bodo, 2.

8   Kenneth C. Haugk, *Christian Caregiving: A Way of Life.* (Minneapolis: Augsburg Publishing House, 1984),19.

9   Haugk, 21.

### 13 Confronting Rejection and Loneliness

1. Temple Grandin, "Needs of High Functioning Teenagers and Adults with Autism: Tips from a Recovered Autistic" in *Focus on Autistic Behavior*, Richard Simpson, ed. Vol. 5, No. 1, April 1990), 8.

2. Henri J.M. Nouwen, *The Inner Voice of Love* (New York: Image Books, 1996), 109.

3. Fredrica R. Halligan, *Listening Deeply to God: Exploring Spirituality in an Interreligious Age* (Toronto: Novalis, 2003), 14.

4. Jean Vanier, *Our Journey Home* (Ottawa: Novalis, 1997), 129.

5. Viktor E. Frankl, "From Experiences in a Concentration Camp" in *Pilgrim Souls: A Collection of Spiritual Autobiographies*, Amy Mandelker and Elizabeth Powers, eds. (Chicago: Franciscan Herald Press, 1983), 494.

6. Murray Bodo, *The Way of St. Francis: The Challenge of Franciscan Spirituality for Everyone* (Cincinnati, OH: St. Anthony Messenger Press, 1995), 135.

### 14 Pilgrims' Process

1. Murray Bodo, *The Way of St. Francis: The Challenge of Franciscan Spirituality for Everyone* (Cincinnati, OH: St. Anthony Messenger Press, 1995), 69–70.

2. Murray Bodo, *The Place We Call Home: Spiritual Pilgrimage as a Path to God* (Brewster, MA: Paraclete Press, 2004), 28–29.

3. V.C. Keating, *The Fire Stone* (Victoria, BC: Trafford, 2004), 152.

4. Catherine de Hueck Doherty, *Poustinia* (Combermere, ON: Madonna House Publications, 1993), 67.

5. Bodo, *The Place We Call Home*, 27.

6. *The Asian Journal of Thomas Merton*. Edited from his original notebooks by Naomi Burton, Brother Patrick Hart and James Laughlin. Consulting editor: Amiya Chakravarty. (New York: A New Directions Book, 1973), 350.

# About the Authors

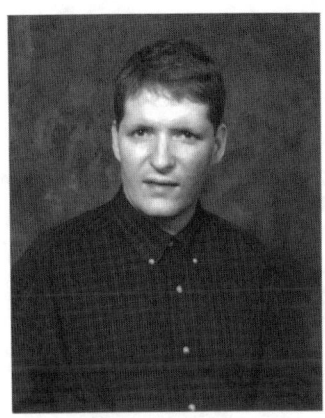

**J. Kevin Vasey** is interested in world events, social justice, travel, nature and music. He is exceptionally sensitive to the plight of persons who suffer injustice, whether it be for reasons of race, culture, religion or disability. Kevin, who has autism and communicates through a Dynavox computer, hopes to exert a positive influence in the world.

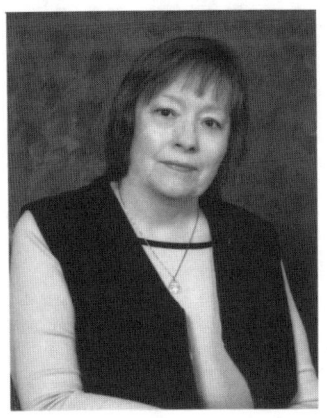

**Gloria Pearson-Vasey**, who has been a Secular Franciscan for 20 years, has a Master of Divinity degree and a background in nursing, music and journalism. A wife, mother and grandmother, she is a pastoral minister and volunteers with individuals who have autism.